Type 1 Diabetes - Causes, Treatments and Management

Edited by Ruxing Zhao

Published in London, United Kingdom

Type 1 Diabetes - Causes, Treatments and Management
http://dx.doi.org/10.5772/intechopen.1003468
Edited by Ruxing Zhao

Contributors
Adebola Busola Ojo, Adriana Gherbon, AliReza Lotfi, Emmanuel Henry Ezenabor, Fatemeh Pournaghi Azar, Issa Rasheed Fetian, Jun Qin, Lukas Villiger, Majid Mobasseri, Mohseen, Morteza Ghojazadeh, Muzaffer Serdar Deniz, Oluwafemi Adeleke Ojo, Rajesh Kumar Sharma, Ruxing Zhao, Sagar Acharya, Sanchari Bhattacharyya, Stefan Zechmann, Tenifayo Soyinka, Tixiao Wang, Wenjing Meng, Yashika Saini

First published in London, United Kingdom, 2025 by IntechOpen
IntechOpen is the global imprint of INTECHOPEN LIMITED, registered in England and Wales, registration number: 11086078, 167-169 Great Portland Street, London, W1W 5PF, United Kingdom

For EU product safety concerns: IN TECH d.o.o., Prolaz Marije Krucifikse Kozulić 3, 51000 Rijeka, Croatia, info@intechopen.com or visit our website at intechopen.com.

British Library Cataloguing-in-Publication Data
A catalogue record for this book is available from the British Library

Type 1 Diabetes - Causes, Treatments and Management
Edited by Ruxing Zhao
p. cm.
Print ISBN 978-1-83769-970-4
Online ISBN 978-1-83769-969-8
eBook (PDF) ISBN 978-1-83769-971-1

Meet the editor

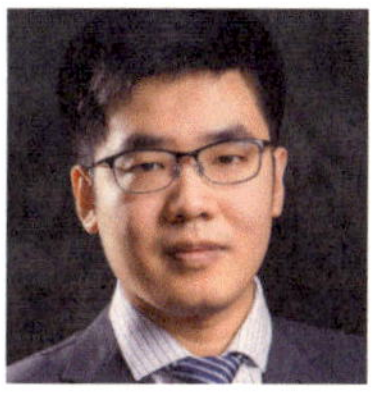

Dr. Ruxing Zhao is now an Associate Chief Physician and Associate Research Professor at Qilu Hospital of Shandong University, as well as an Associate Professor at Shandong University. He also serves as the Deputy Director of the Shandong Provincial Key Laboratory of Temporal Regulation and Precision Intervention in Endocrine and Metabolic Diseases. His research focuses on the role of immune-inflammatory mechanisms in endocrine and metabolic diseases, particularly how environmental factors (gut microbiota, diet, and lifestyle) influence glucose and lipid metabolism through immunometabolism circadian rhythms and epigenetic regulation. Dr. Zhao has developed practical tools for assessing pancreatic β-cell function and contributed to the improvement of endocrine function tests.

Contents

Preface

The management of diabetes has been identified as a formidable challenge within the global public health landscape of the 21st century. Type 1 Diabetes Mellitus (T1DM) has emerged as a pivotal subtype, characterized by the immune-mediated destruction of β-cells. Despite remarkable advancements in understanding its pathogenesis, therapeutic interventions, and management strategies, T1DM continues to exert a significant burden on patients, healthcare systems, and society at large. Recently, groundbreaking advancements in immunological research, innovative therapeutic modalities, and the burgeoning field of digital health have begun to revolutionize the paradigm of T1DM management.

This treatise is meant to serve as an encyclopedic reference for clinicians, researchers, and public health practitioners. It encompasses both foundational theories and clinical applications, as well as traditional diagnostic and treatment methods alongside cutting-edge technologies, all in pursuit of enhancing comprehensive T1DM lifecycle management. Our goal is to provide an extensive professional resource that not only systematically consolidates the existing knowledge base but also focuses on the latest advancements and future directions in the science and clinical management of T1DM.

This volume is designed to provide scholars and researchers in the fields of immunology, metabolism, and biomedical engineering with the latest advancements in the study of T1DM. It provides a comprehensive discussion of the pathogenesis, pathophysiology, and therapeutic strategies relevant to T1DM. The text delves into the mechanisms underpinning T1DM, elucidating transformative opportunities, clarifying unresolved challenges, and charting pathways for future inquiry. This provides strategic guidance for ongoing research. Simultaneously, this treatise caters to clinicians, including endocrinologists, diabetologists, pediatricians, and general practitioners, by synthesizing evidence-based medicine and systematically integrating the knowledge base from the spectrum of T1DM, from pathogenesis to long-term management. It facilitates the translation of fundamental and cutting-edge research findings, fostering a union between clinical practice and basic research.

Furthermore, the volume addresses the psychosocial dimensions of T1DM, guiding patients in cultivating psychological resilience and enhancing social adaptability. It also serves as a reference for public health professionals engaged in the formulation of diabetes prevention and control policies. This book distinguishes itself by combining interdisciplinary perspectives, offering researchers in the fields of medicine and artificial intelligence, as well as readers interested in this convergent field, a comprehensive vantage point. By integrating cutting-edge technologies such as artificial intelligence-assisted diagnostics and predictive analytics based on big data into the traditional corpus of medical knowledge, it constructs a holistic management framework for T1DM that unites biology, medicine, society, and technology. Within its pages, readers will gain an in-depth understanding of the application of data science in medical diagnosis and healthcare services management, inspiring insights that may catalyze their own research or professional endeavours.

In the wake of significant advancements, the field of T1DM continues to grapple with numerous unmet clinical needs. This book not only systematically consolidates extant research findings but also delves into pivotal issues: precision medicine tailored to individual immunometabolic profiles, sophisticated smart closed-loop systems designed to alleviate the burden of patient management, innovative strides in disease-modifying strategies encompassing the induction of immune tolerance and regenerative medicine, and global collaborative scientific endeavors aimed at accelerating the realization of fundamental therapeutic breakthroughs for T1DM. Within the etiology section, an exhaustive examination of the pathogenic origins of T1DM is provided, examining both genetic and environmental factors, elucidating the interplay among these elements, and unveiling the scientific mechanisms underlying this complex disease. The epidemiology segment provides an in-depth analysis of global epidemiological data for T1DM, including trend evaluations of incidence and prevalence, offering a comprehensive perspective on the disease's occurrence, evolutionary trajectory, and demographic variations worldwide. This enables readers to grasp the macro-level distribution characteristics of the condition. The pathophysiology chapter meticulously expounds upon the pathological processes of T1DM, covering autoimmune mechanisms, the degradation and attrition of pancreatic beta cells, the latest advancements in beta cell dynamics research, the decline in insulin secretion, and the resultant systemic metabolic dysregulation. This provides a comprehensive depiction of the physiological changes intrinsic to the disease. The treatment and management section systematically introduces therapeutic strategies for T1DM, encompassing insulin therapy, blood glucose monitoring, dietary control, exercise guidance, and the prevention and management of complications, with an emphasis on the significance of integrative treatment. The sociopsychological chapter focuses on the mental state of patients with T1DM, discussing the psychological impact of the disease on the patients and their families, and highlighting the role of psychological interventions and social support in aiding patients in coping with their illness. Finally, the chapter on recent research progress outlines the cutting-edge scientific advancements in the field of T1DM, including novel therapies, immune regulation, stem cell treatments, genetic therapies, and disease prevention. It also discusses the application of data science and artificial intelligence in the realm of diabetes and their potential to enhance the quality of healthcare and construct efficient healthcare systems. Additionally, the book introduces high-performance bioinformatics data analysis and processing models and methods developed for the characteristics of bio-medical health data (multi-source, heterogeneous, dynamic, massive), facilitating their application in diabetes prediction, diagnosis, complication screening, and blood glucose management by clinicians, and delineating future directions for disease research.

In compiling this comprehensive volume, we have leveraged the aggregated expertise and support of a multitude of colleagues. We extend our deepest appreciation to our editorial team, with whom we have collaboratively achieved the culmination of this scholarly endeavor. We also hold in high esteem the intrepid clinical professionals at the forefront, who have generously contributed their precious case studies and experiences. Our gratitude is also directed towards our family, whose unwavering understanding and support serve as our perpetual motivation. Moreover, we are sincerely thankful to the T1DM patients who selflessly shared their personal experiences, whose narratives have profoundly resonated with us and steadfastly strengthened our dedication to providing exemplary care to patients. We extend our profound gratitude to all the scholars whose works have been referenced in the present paper, as well as to the investigators in contiguous disciplines whose erudite contributions have bolstered the scholarly underpinnings of this research endeavor. Additionally, we extend our heartfelt appreciation for the comprehensive informational resources provided by the library and the digital reading room.

This volume is a tribute to the scholarly acumen and steadfast dedication of scientific investigators, clinical specialists, and the resilient patient cohort united in their quest to advance the understanding of T1DM. It is compiled to serve as an authoritative compendium within the professional domain, with the aspiration that it will kindle a surge of innovative ingenuity, driving us toward the audacious objective of eradicating T1DM from our global community.

Should any queries or recommendations arise during the examination of this book, please do not hesitate to contact us through our formal communication channels. This will enable us to provide the requisite support and feedback expeditiously and precisely.

Ruxing Zhao
Department of Endocrinology and Metabolism,
Qilu Hospital of Shandong University,
Shandong Provincial Key Laboratory of Spatiotemporal Regulation
and Precision Intervention in Endocrine and Metabolic Diseases,
Jinan, China

Section 1

Fundamentals and Epidemiology

Chapter 1

Epidemiology of Type 1 Diabetes

Adriana Gherbon

Abstract

The prevalence of diabetes mellitus is increasing globally. In 2021, 537 million people have diabetes, and this number will be 643 million by 2030 and 783 million by 2045. In 2021, more than 6.7 million people aged 20–79 died from diabetes-related causes. The number of children and adolescents (up to 19 years old) living with diabetes continues to rise each year. In 2021, it was estimated that over 1.2 million children and adolescents were living with type 1 diabetes. Direct healthcare costs related to diabetes are extremely high, reaching approximately one trillion USD in 2021, and are expected to surpass this figure by 2030.

Keywords: prevalence, type 1 diabetes, gender, age, country

1. Introduction

Knowledge of the epidemiological data, regarding the evolutionary trends of diabetes mellitus (DM), is necessary to ensure a rational health policy, to identify individuals, groups or communities at high risk of developing this condition, as well as to elucidate the etiopathogenesis of DM and implement some effective primary, secondary and tertiary prevention programs.

The main parameters monitored to assess the frequency of DM and its complications are [1]:

- *Prevalence*: the total number of existing cases at a given time in a certain area; it is expressed as a proportion (%), being dependent on the frequency of the appearance of new cases and their lifetime;

- *Incidence*: the number of new cases/100,000 people observed in a period of time, usually one year;

- *Incidence rate*: the ratio between the number of new cases of the disease in a certain area diagnosed in a certain time period and the number of non-diabetic subjects in the same region in the same time interval;

- *Cumulative incidence*: the sum of annual incidences over a period of time. At young ages, it overlaps with prevalence. At older ages, however, the prevalence of the disease will be lower than the cumulative incidence because, over time, some patients have died.

Although DM has been known since Antiquity, actual epidemiological data only exists from the first half of the last century. The "modern" epidemiology of DM began about 50 years ago through the first population study conducted in Sudbury (USA) [2]. A landmark for the continuation of epidemiological research in the field of DM is the publication by West (1978) of the work "Epidemiology of diabetes and its vascular complications" [3].

Epidemiological studies carried out up to the 1980s do not allow direct comparisons of reported prevalence with current data due to the lack of standardized diagnostic and case-recording methodologies up to that date. In addition, the change in diagnostic criteria for DM in 1999 amplifies this problem by directly influencing epidemiological data.

Currently, there is an impressive dynamic of increasing the prevalence of DM worldwide.

2. Epidemiological data

DM type 1 is one of the most common chronic diseases of children and adolescents, but it can also occur in adults and represents 5–10% of all DM cases.

In 2021, it was estimated that around 8.4 million people worldwide were living with type 1 diabetes (T1DM), with 500,000 new cases reported that year. By 2040, the global number of individuals living with T1DM is expected to rise to between 13.5 and 17.4 million [4].

Epidemiological data about T1DM are different in children and adolescents compared to adults.

2.1 Epidemiological data for children and adolescents

In the past, the most important data currently available regarding the epidemiology of DM type 1 in children (0–14 years) were provided by the EURO-DIAB-ACE [5] and WHO-Dia Mond (the Multinational Project for Childhood diabetes) [6] studies, initiated in 1989 and 1990, respectively.

The incidence and prevalence estimates of type 1 diabetes in children and adolescents (ages 0–14 and 0–19) were provided by the 10th Edition of the IDF Diabetes Atlas Type 1 Diabetes in Children and Adolescents Special Interest Group [7]. According to this atlas, the total number of children and adolescents aged 0–19 living with type 1 diabetes is 1.2 million, with 184,100 new diagnoses each year [7].

The incidence and prevalence of T1DM are increasing each year due to rising incidence in many countries [8] and reductions in mortality. It is estimated that globally, the total number of children and adolescents with T1DM is 1,211,900, and around 108,200 children and adolescents under 15 years are diagnosed each year. When we consider the persons more than 20 years this number rises to 149,500 [7].

Global estimates for type 1 diabetes in children and adolescents (0–14 years and 0–19 years) in 2021, according to IDF Atlas 10th edition, are written in **Table 1** [7]:

It has been observed that the highest incidence rates are found in populations of Northern European descent, as well as in countries from the Middle East and North Africa [9]. Among the ten countries with the highest incidence rates, four are now from non-European regions. A recent report from Eritrea highlighted a particularly high incidence in migrant populations from this area of Africa, specifically in the 15–24-year age group [10].

	Global population	Number of prevalent (existing) cases of type 1 diabetes	Number of incident (new) cases of type 1 diabetes per year
Type 1 diabetes in children and adolescents (0–14 years)	1.99 billion	651,700	108,300
Type 1 diabetes in children and adolescents (0–19 years)	2.61 billion	1,211,900	149,500

Table 1.
Global estimates for type 1 diabetes in children and adolescents (0–14 years and 0–19 years) in 2021 according to IDF Atlas 10th edition.

In **Figure 1** are listed the top 10 countries or territories with the highest estimated number of new (incident) cases of type 1 diabetes in children and adolescents (ages 0–19) per year, according to the 10th edition of the IDF Atlas [7].

Regarding the prevalence of T1DM in the EUR and NAC regions is the highest number of prevalent cases due to high incidence rates.

Compared to the previous years, larger discrepancies were found for Mali [11], the Maldives [12], and Canada [13, 14], probably because of rapid changes in mortality, diagnosed incidence, and differences between regions within countries.

The highest prevalence of T1DM in people under 20 years of age is in India (229,400), followed by the USA (157,900) and Brazil 92,300.

The first 10 countries or territories with the highest estimated number of prevalent (existing) cases of type 1 diabetes in children and adolescents (0–19 years) per annum according to IDF Atlas 10th edition [7] are:

- India - 229,400
- United States of America - 157,900
- Brazil - 92,300
- China - 56,000
- Algeria - 50,800
- Morocco - 43,300
- Russian Federation - 38,100
- Germany - 35,100
- United Kingdom - 31,600
- Saudi Arabia - 28,900

2.2 Epidemiological data for adult-onset type 1 diabetes

T1DM is common in children and adolescents, but it can also be present in adults. Frequently, it is misdiagnosed as type 2 diabetes, leading to an underestimation of the adult-onset type 1 diabetes.

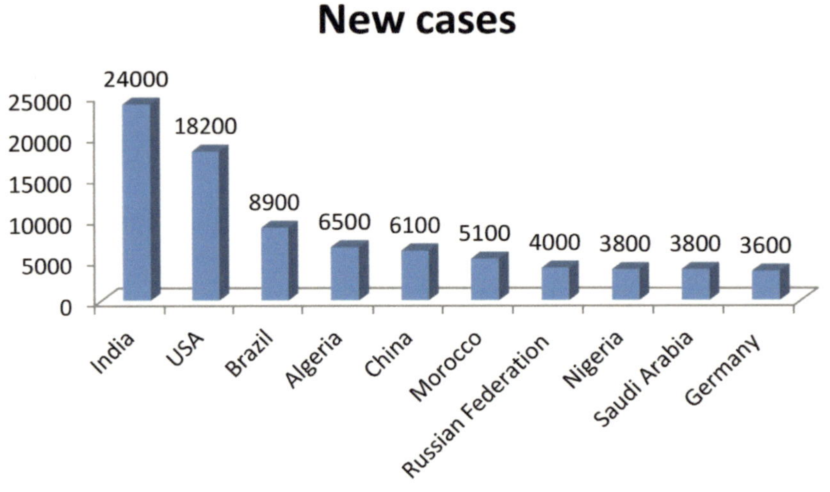

Figure 1.
The top 10 countries or territories with the highest estimated number of new (incident) cases of type 1 diabetes in children and adolescents (ages 0–19) per year, according to the 10th edition of the IDF Atlas.

The highest incidence of adult-onset type 1 diabetes is in Eritrea with 46.2/100,000/year and the lowest in Spain with 9.9/100,000/year. It was observed that countries with higher incidence of T1DM in children and adolescents have also higher incidence of T1DM in adults [7]. The studies showed that the incidence of adult-onset type 1 diabetes is, in general, higher among men than women and did not decline with increasing age, remaining substantial across the life course [15].

The first 10 countries with the highest incidence of adult-onset type 1 diabetes according to IDF Atlas 10th edition [7] are:

- Eritrea (study year 2019) - 46.2/100,000
- Sweden (study year 2009) - 30.6/100,000
- Ireland (study year 2011–2016) - 30.6/100,000
- Finland (study year 2017) - 24/100,000
- United KIngdom (study year 2009–2013) - 17.8/100,000
- Norway (study year 1978–1982) - 16.7/100,000
- United States (study year 2017) - 16.5/100,000
- Australia (study year 2020) - 16.4/100,000
- Libia (study year 1981–1990) - 9.9/100,000
- Spain (study year 1987–1990) - 9.9/100,000

The incidence of type 1 DM shows great variability over time, depending on age, sex, race, ethnicity, and geographic location.

3. Variability of T1DM incidence

3.1 Temporal changes in the incidence of DM type 1

Data on the incidence of type 1 DM over time is indicative and useful for testing its various pathogenic hypotheses. The absence of large variations in incidence from one generation to another is a characteristic feature of a pure genetic disease. If there are important variations in it, the aspect pleads for the intervention of environmental factors in the pathogenesis of DM type 1. Until the last two decades, DM type 1 was considered to be a stable condition in terms of incidence and individual risk, but recent epidemiological studies have demonstrated an increasing trend in its incidence on all continents, in all ethnic groups, and at all ages [16].

This increasing incidence can probably be related to some environmental factors, still uncertain (excessive pollution, viral infections, reduced breastfeeding of infants and early exposure to cow's milk proteins, toxic substances, low zinc intake, vitamin D deficiency, etc.), because the time interval is too short to incriminate an increase in genetic susceptibility to the disease [16].

3.2 Seasonal variability in the incidence of DM type 1

The existence of a seasonal variation in the incidence of DM type 1 was found, in the sense that, in the cold months of the year (winter, autumn, early spring), more cases are diagnosed than in the warm seasons [17]. This seasonal trend is more evident in older children, during puberty, respectively in populations at increased risk for DM. In low-incidence countries, seasonal variation could not be proven, sometimes the reverse phenomenon could be observed (more cases recorded in summer than in winter).

Because pancreatic β-cell destruction usually begins several years before the clinical onset of the disease, the seasonal occurrence of new cases reflects, in particular, seasonal variations in individual susceptibility to various precipitating environmental factors. Another explanation could be a higher incidence of infections at lower temperatures and increased humidity and, hypothetically, the triggering of autoimmune processes [18].

3.3 Variations in the incidence of DM type 1 according to age and sex

In previous European studies, the age of children with the highest incidence was between 0 and 4 years [19, 20]. The study from Finland showed a significant decrease in the incidence of T1DM in children younger than 7 years of age but less in older children. Also, a rise in the median age at diagnosis was found, more prominent in boys [21].

The highest and lowest incidences of T1DM in children aged 5–9 and 10–14 years are listed in **Table 2**.

Recent studies indicate that more adults than children are diagnosed with T1DM each year (316,000 vs. 194,000 incident cases globally in 2021), with an average diagnosis age of 32 years [23]. Additionally, there appears to be an age-dependent pattern of T1DM incidence, with the incidence increasing as age rises [24].

Autoimmune diseases, including T1DM, are more frequently diagnosed in females [25]. However, some studies show a predominance of T1DM in males, with

Incidence of T1DM	5–9 years	10–14 years
Highest		
Northern Africa	44.78/100,000 per year	40.92/100,000 per year
Northern Europe	37.17/100,000 per year	41.48/100,000 per year
Northern America	26.31/100,000 per year	33.50/100,000 per year
Lowest		
Southern Asia	0.92/100,000 per year	1.99/100,000 per year
Eastern Asia	1.93/100,000 per year	2.78/100,000 per year
South America	4.47/100,000 per year	3.62/100,000 per year

Table 2.
The highest and lowest incidence of T1DM in children aged 5–9 and 10–14 years [22].

differences emerging after puberty [26]. Generally, populations with higher incidences of T1DM tend to show a greater male predominance. For example, in some European countries, the incidence of T1DM is higher in boys than in girls, while in some Asian countries, a higher incidence is seen in girls [26–28].

Because genetic factors alone cannot explain the rapid increase in T1DM incidence, various environmental and socioeconomic factors have been implicated. Recent research has pointed to early life factors, including maternal diet, mode of delivery, infant feeding, childhood diet, microbial exposure, and air pollution, all of which may impact the development of T1DM in early childhood [16].

3.4 Other factors influencing the incidence of T1DM

3.4.1 Gestational age

Research has shown a link between gestational age, birth weight, and the risk of Type 1 Diabetes Mellitus (T1DM). Children born with a low birth weight (less than 2500 g) have a higher likelihood of developing T1DM. Potential mechanisms for this may include insulin resistance due to fetal growth restriction or changes in gut microbiota [29]. On the other hand, data on the risk associated with a birth weight over 4000 g is conflicting [30, 31].

3.4.2 Cesarean section

The relationship between cesarean section (CS) and the diagnosis of T1DM remains inconclusive. However, recent studies suggest that delivery by CS does not increase the risk of developing T1DM [32, 33].

3.4.3 Maternal age

Maternal age has also been suggested as a potential risk factor for T1DM. A 2010 meta-analysis found a weak but significant linear rise in T1DM risk with increasing maternal age. However, it concluded that only a small portion of the recent rise in T1DM incidence can be attributed to this factor [34].

3.4.4 Puberty

Puberty has been linked to an increased incidence of T1DM [35]. The proposed mechanism is insulin resistance during puberty, even in non-diabetic individuals, which leads to the worsening of fasting and postprandial insulin levels, along with excessive growth hormone (GH) secretion [35].

3.5 Geographical variations in the incidence of type 1 DM

One of the most important features of type 1 DM is the great geographic variability in the incidence of cases. Thus, a variability is found:

- *Intercontinental*: **Table 3**.
- *Between the two hemispheres*: incidence rates are higher in the northern hemisphere than in the southern hemisphere;
- *Within the same hemisphere*: there is a north/south gradient of type DM incidence;
- *Intracontinental*: in addition to the north–south gradient, in Europe we can also speak of a west/east or, rather, northwest/southeast gradient;
- *Within the same country*: in China, the coefficient of variation is about 50:1 between Zunyi 0.1/100000 and Wuhan 4.6/100000, two Chinese provinces; in Sardinia, the incidence of DM type 1 is 3–5 times higher than in mainland Italy [1].

The variability within the same country was partly explained by the ethnic heterogeneity of the population, although marked variations were also observed in countries that have a relatively homogeneous population from a genetic point of view: Finland, Sweden, and Norway.

Because it is not known whether this huge geographic variability in type 1 DM incidence is caused by differences in genetic susceptibility, by variations in the distribution of environmental determinants, or by their combination, future

Incidence of T1DM	Highest	Lowest
0–14 years	*Northern Europe* 23.96 per 100,000 *Australia/New Zealand* 22.8 per 100,000 *Northern America* 18.02 per 100,000	*Melanesia* *Western Africa* *South America* all <1 per 100,000
0–19 years	*Northern Europe* 39.0 per 100,000 *Northern America* 20.07 per 100,000 *Northern Africa* 10.1 per 100,000	*Eastern Africa* *Western Africa* all <2 per 100,000

Table 3.
The intercontinental variability of type 1 DM [22].

epidemiological research will attempt to explain this phenomenon and, related to it, to find effective prophylactic methods.

3.6 Racial and ethnic variations in the incidence of type 1 DM

If there are racial and ethnic differences in the risk of type 1 DM within the same population, they are not as important as geographic differences. Thus, in the US, the non-Hispanic white population has a 1.5 times greater risk of developing type 1 DM compared to African Americans or the Hispanic population. Immigrants from Germany (Italians, Greeks, Turks) have the same risk for DM as the population from the country of origin, Hungarians from Romania have a higher risk for DM type 1, compared to Romanians (risk close to that registered in Hungary). The hypothesis was thus drawn that ethnic groups seem to retain their genetic susceptibility, regardless of the country in which they live [1].

Contrary to these observations, it is interesting that emigrants from a country with a low incidence of type 1 DM will acquire a risk of DM similar to that of the population in the country in which they live (e.g., children from South Asia who immigrated to the Great Britain); in these cases, environmental factors seem to play a decisive role [1].

4. Prevalence of T1DM complications

Type 1 diabetes (T1D) is associated with several complications that can significantly impact health. The prevalence of these complications varies based on factors such as disease duration, glycemic control, and individual health conditions.

4.1 Acute complications

Diabetic Ketoacidosis (DKA) affects 4.6–8.0 per 1000 individuals with diabetes each year [36]. The incidence is higher among those with type 1 diabetes, with approximately 4% of people in the United Kingdom developing DKA annually, compared to 25% in Malaysia [37, 38]. In the United States, DKA leads to 135,000 hospital admissions each year [39]. Around 30% of children are diagnosed with type 1 diabetes after experiencing an episode of DKA [40]. Additionally, lower socioeconomic status and greater area-level deprivation are linked to a higher risk of DKA in individuals with type 1 diabetes [41].

Once thought to be universally fatal, the risk of death from diabetic ketoacidosis (DKA) with proper and timely treatment is now between <1% and 5% [37, 42]. Up to 1% of children with DKA experience a complication called cerebral edema [43]. In the United States, the incidence of cerebral edema in children with DKA has increased from 0.4% in 2002 to 0.7% in 2012 [44]. Between 2 and 5 out of 10 children who develop brain swelling will die as a result [45]. Ketoacidosis is responsible for 13–19% of deaths related to type 1 diabetes, [37] making it the leading cause of death among people with type 1 diabetes under the age of 58 [38].

4.2 Hypoglycemia

In individuals with poor glycemic control, the annual incidence of severe hypoglycemia can reach as high as 8.3%. On average, people with type 1 diabetes experience two mild, symptomatic episodes of hypoglycemia per week [46]. Additionally, those with type 1 diabetes will have at least one severe hypoglycemic episode per year that requires assistance [46]. On average, individuals with type 1 diabetes experience a hypoglycemia event requiring help 16–20 times per 100 person-years and an event that leads to unconsciousness or a seizure 2–8 times per 100 person-years [47]. In terms of mortality, hypoglycemia is responsible for 6–10% of deaths among individuals with type 1 diabetes [46].

4.3 Chronic complications

Diabetic Retinopathy (DR) is a major cause of vision impairment in individuals with type 1 diabetes (T1D), affecting about 28% of patients. Overall, around 35% of people with diabetes have some form of diabetic retinopathy, with 10% experiencing some degree of vision loss [48]. DR is particularly prevalent in those with type 1 diabetes, impacting 25% of individuals five years after diagnosis, 60% after 10 years, and 80% after 15 years [49]. The progression of the disease is largely influenced by blood sugar management, with about 7% of individuals with diabetes developing proliferative diabetic retinopathy and 7% experiencing diabetic macular edema [48]. Diabetic retinopathy remains the leading cause of vision loss among individuals aged 20–74 [48].

Diabetic Nephropathy (DN) is a major contributor to end-stage renal disease (ESRD). The incidence of ESRD due to diabetes is approximately 2.2% 20 years after diagnosis. About one-third of individuals with type 1 and type 2 diabetes are affected by diabetic nephropathy. This condition is responsible for roughly one-third of ESRD cases globally, with an even higher proportion in developed countries [50]. The progression of diabetic kidney disease can lead to ESRD and an increased risk of cardiovascular complications, both of which contribute to a significant economic burden [51]. In developed nations, certain ethnic groups, such as African Americans and Native Americans, face a higher risk of developing diabetic nephropathy and ESRD [52].

4.4 Cardiovascular diseases (CVD)

People with T1D also have a higher risk of cardiovascular disease, which is estimated to shorten their lifespan by 8–13 years [47]. Additionally, women with type 1 diabetes are 40% more likely to die compared to men with the condition [53].

4.5 Neuropathy

A systematic review has revealed that diabetic peripheral neuropathy impacts 30% of individuals with diabetes [54]. Additionally, diabetic neuropathy is responsible for 50–75% of non-traumatic amputations.

The primary risk factor for diabetic neuropathy is hyperglycemia. In the Diabetes Control and Complications Trial (DCCT) of 1995, the annual incidence of neuropathy was 2% per year, but this reduced to 0.56% with intensive treatment in individuals with type 1 diabetes. The progression of neuropathy is closely linked to glycemic control in both type 1 and type 2 diabetes. Additional risk factors include the duration of diabetes, age, smoking, hypertension, height, and hyperlipidemia [54].

5. Prevalence of T1DM comorbidities

5.1 Celiac disease

In children with type 1 diabetes mellitus (T1DM), the incidence of celiac disease is elevated, ranging from 0.6% to 16.4% [55]. Studies indicate that the prevalence of celiac disease in children with diabetes is 20 times higher than in the general population [56]. In approximately 90% of cases, celiac disease develops after the onset of T1DM and is typically identified through screening tests. It is rare for celiac disease to be diagnosed before diabetes [57, 58]. Risk factors for developing celiac disease in individuals with T1DM include being female and having an early diagnosis of diabetes [55, 59].

5.2 Autoimmune gastritis

In individuals with T1DM, the prevalence of APCA ranges from 3–30% (with a rate of 5.3–7.2% in children and adolescents) [60–62]. In contrast, the prevalence among healthy children aged 0–15 years is much lower, between 0.3% and 1.98% [60, 62, 63].

The possible mechanism of association between these two diseases is the presence of GAD antigen in the pancreas, but also in the gastric mucosa and submucosa. The response of T cells to the GAD antigen begins in the pancreas, and then the autoimmune process expands, destroying other neuroendocrine tissues [64].

5.3 Addison disease

T1DM in children and adolescents typically occurs before the onset of AD [65], which has an incidence rate of about 1–2% in adult T1DM patients. Conversely, the incidence of T1DM among patients with AD ranges from 10–18% [66]. Type 1 diabetes is most commonly seen in patients with PAS-1 and PAS-2.

5.4 Vitiligo

The incidence of vitiligo in the general population is between 0.5% and 1% [67], with more than 50% of cases being diagnosed before the age of 20 [68]. Vitiligo may occur prior to the development of T1DM [69], and approximately 16–20% of vitiligo patients may develop diabetes. Polyglandular autoimmune syndrome PAS-2 often begins with the onset of vitiligo [70], which is more common in individuals with T1DM [71].

5.5 Thyroid disorders

People with type 1 diabetes are at an increased risk for developing several autoimmune disorders, particularly thyroid problems – around 20% of people with type 1 diabetes have hypothyroidism or hyperthyroidism, typically caused by Hashimoto's thyroiditis or Graves' disease, respectively [64].

5.6 PAS

The incidence of type 1 diabetes in these syndromes is 4–18% in PAS-1, 60% in PAS-2, and 14.5% in PAS-3. While clinical symptoms typically emerge in the third decade of life, the initial signs can appear during childhood. As a result, it is crucial for pediatricians to be familiar with the symptoms of PAS, particularly in the context of multiple autoimmune comorbidities associated with type 1 diabetes [66, 72].

5.7 Organ-nonspecific autoimmune diseases

In patients with type 1 diabetes, organ-nonspecific autoimmune diseases can develop, such as juvenile idiopathic arthritis (JIA), Sjögren's syndrome, or psoriasis [72, 73]. However, there is limited research on these T1DM comorbidities, especially in pediatric patients [72].

6. Conclusions

In conclusion, we can say that we can talk about diabetes in terms of an "epidemic." Its prevalence at the global level is constantly increasing, even if in recent years there are some countries that have reported a slight reduction in the growth rate of its incidence of forecasts. DM remains a very important medico-social problem because it affects the quality and length of life of patients, having numerous implications of a social, professional, family nature, and beyond.

Health costs related to DM are very high globally, especially due to complications, thus requiring preventive measures (optimization of lifestyle), active detection of the disease, and effective and early treatment.

Conflict of interest

The authors declare no conflict of interest.

Author details

Adriana Gherbon
University of Medicine and Pharmacy "V. Babes", Timisoara, Romania

*Address all correspondence to: gherbon.adriana@umft.ro

References

[1] Botea V, Serban V. Epidemiology of diabetes. In: Serban V, editor. Romanian Treatise on Metabolic Diseases. Brumar Publishing House; 2010. pp. 79-86. ISBN 978-973-602-527-3

[2] O'Sullivan JB, Williams RF. Early diabetes mellitus in perspective: A population study in Sudbury, mass. Journal of the American Medical Association. 1966;**198**(6):579-582. DOI: 10.1001/jama.1966.03110190061018

[3] West K. Epidemiology of Diabetes and its Vascular Complications. New York: Elsevier; 1978

[4] Gregory GA, TIG R, Linklater SE, Wang F, Colagiuri S, de Beaufort C, et al. International diabetes federation diabetes atlas type 1 diabetes in adults special interest group; global incidence, prevalence, and mortality of type 1 diabetes in 2021 with projection to 2040: A modelling study. The Lancet Diabetes and Endocrinology. 2022;**10**(10):741-760. DOI: 10.1016/S2213-8587(22)00218-2

[5] Green A, Gale EA, Patterson CC. Incidence of childhood-onset insulin-dependent diabetes mellitus: The EURODIAB ACE study. Lancet. 1992;**339**(8798):905-909. DOI: 10.1016/0140-6736(92)90938-y

[6] WHO Multinational Project for Childhood Diabetes. WHO diamond project group. Diabetes Care. 1990;**13**(10):1062-1068. DOI: 10.2337/diacare.13.10.1062

[7] Magliano DJ, Boyko EJ. IDF diabetes atlas 10th edition scientific committee. In: IDF Diabetes Atlas [internet]. 10th ed. Brussels: International Diabetes Federation; 2021. Available from: https://www.ncbi.nlm.nih.gov/books/NBK581934/

[8] Tuomilehto J, Ogle GD, Lund-Blix N, Stene LC. Epidemiology of childhood type 1 diabetes. Pediatric Endocrinology Reviews. 2020;**17**(Suppl. 1):198-209. DOI: 10.17458/per.vol17.2020.tol.epidemiologychildtype1diabetes

[9] Ogle GD, James S, Dabelea D, Pihoker C, Svennson J, Maniam J, et al. Global estimates of incidence of type 1 diabetes in children and adolescents: Results from the international diabetes federation atlas, 10th edition. Diabetes Research and Clinical Practice. Jan 2021;**183**:109083. DOI: 10.1016/j.diabres.2021.109083. Epub 2021 Dec 6

[10] Mebrahtu G, Maniam J, James S, Ogle GD. High incidence of type 1 diabetes in adolescents and young adults in Eritrea. Diabetic Medicine. 2021;**15**:e14544. DOI: 10.1111/dme.14544

[11] Sandy JL, Besançon S, Sidibé AT, Minkailou M, Togo A, Ogle GD. Rapid increases in observed incidence and prevalence of type 1 diabetes in children and youth in Mali, 2007-2016. Pediatric Diabetes. 2021;**22**(4):545-551. DOI: 10.1111/pedi.13191

[12] Majeed NA, Shiruhana SA, Maniam J, Eigenmann CA, Siyan A, Ogle GD. Incidence, prevalence and mortality of diabetes in children and adolescents aged under 20 years in the Republic of Maldives. Journal of Paediatrics and Child Health. 2020;**56**:746-750. DOI: 10.1111/jpc.14726

[13] Cummings E, Flemming M, Talbot P. Trends in incidence of type 1 diabetes in children and adolescents over 25 years in Nova Scotia Canada: 1994-2018. Pediatric Diabetes. 2021;**22**(Suppl. 29):EP003. DOI: 10.1111/pedi.13198

[14] Fox DA, Islam N, Sutherland J, Reimer K, Amed S. Type 1 diabetes incidence and prevalence trends in a cohort of Canadian children and youth. Pediatric Diabetes. 2018;**19**(3):501-505. DOI: 10.1016/j.jpeds.2020.02.069

[15] Harding JL, Wander PL, Zhang X, Li X, Karuranga S, Chen H, et al. The incidence of adult-onset type 1 diabetes: A systematic review from 32 countries and regions. Diabetes Care. 2022;**45**(4):994-1006. DOI: 10.2337/dc21-1752

[16] Ogrotis I, Koufakis T, Kotsa K. Changes in the global epidemiology of type 1 diabetes in an evolving landscape of environmental factors: Causes, challenges, and opportunities. Medicina (Kaunas, Lithuania). 2023;**59**(4):668. DOI: 10.3390/medicina59040668

[17] Turtinen M, Härkönen T, Ilonen J, Parkkola A, Knip M. Finish Pediatric diabetes register. Seasonality in the manifestation of type 1 diabetes varies according to age at diagnosis in Finnish children. Acta Paediatrica. 2022;**111**(5):1061-1069. DOI: 10.1111/apa.16282

[18] Oikarinen S et al. Virus antibody survey in different European populations indicates risk association between coxsackievirus B1 and type 1 diabetes. Diabetes. 2014;**63**:655-662

[19] Patterson CC, Dahlquist GG, Gyürüs E, et al. Incidence trends for childhood type 1 diabetes in Europe during 1989-2003 and predicted new cases 2005-20: A multicentre prospective registration study. Lancet. 2009;**373**:2027-2033. DOI: 10.1016/S0140-6736(09)60568-7

[20] Gardner SG, Bingley PJ, Sawtell PA, et al. Rising incidence of insulin dependent diabetes in children aged under 5 years in the Oxford region: Time trend analysis, The Bart's-Oxford Study Group. BMJ. 1997;**315**:713-717. DOI: 10.1136/BMJ.315.7110.713

[21] Parviainen A, But A, Siljander H, et al. Decreased incidence of type 1 diabetes in young Finnish children. Diabetes Care. 2020;**43**:2953-2958. DOI: 10.2337/DC20-0604

[22] Gomber A, Ward ZJ, Ross C, et al. Variation in the incidence of type 1 diabetes mellitus in children and adolescents by world region and country income group: A scoping review. PLOS Global Public Health. 2022;**2**:e0001099. DOI: 10.1371/JOURNAL.PGPH.0001099

[23] Gregory GA, Robinson TIG, Linklater SE, et al. Global incidence, prevalence, and mortality of type 1 diabetes in 2021 with projection to 2040: A modelling study. The Lancet Diabetes and Endocrinology. 2022;**10**:741-760. DOI: 10.1016/S2213-8587(22)00218-2

[24] Niechciał E, Michalak M, Skowrońska B, et al. Increasing trend of childhood type 1 diabetes incidence: 20-year observation from greater Poland Province, Poland. Acta Diabetologica. 2024;**61**:1609-1617. DOI: 10.1007/s00592-024-02339-5

[25] Angum F, Khan T, Kaler J et al. The Prevalence of Autoimmune Disorders in Women: A Narrative Review; 2020. DOI:10.7759/CUREUS.8094.Cureus 12

[26] Fernández-Ramos C, Arana-Arri E, Jiménez-Huertas P, et al. Incidence of childhood-onset type 1 diabetes in Biscay, Spain, 1990-2013. Pediatric Diabetes. 2017;**18**:71-76. DOI: 10.1111/PEDI.1235

[27] Harjutsalo V, Sund R, Knip M, Groop PH. Incidence of type 1 diabetes

in Finland. JAMA. 2013;**310**:427-428. DOI: 10.1001/JAMA.2013.8399

[28] Kida K, Mimura G, Ito T, et al. Incidence of type 1 diabetes mellitus in children aged 0-14 in Japan, 1986-1990, including an analysis for seasonality of onset and month of birth: JDS study, The Data Committee for Childhood Diabetes of the Japan Diabetes Society (JDS). Diabetic Medicine. 2000;**17**:59-63. DOI: 10.1046/J.1464-5491.2000.00205

[29] Li S et al. Preterm birth and risk of type 1 and type 2 diabetes: Systematic review and meta-analysis. Obesity Reviews. 2014;**15**:804-811

[30] Harder T et al. Birth weight, early weight gain, and subsequent risk of type 1 diabetes: Systematic review and meta-analysis. American Journal of Epidemiology. 2009;**169**:1428-1436

[31] Khasan AS et al. Gestational age and birth weight and the risk of childhood type 1 diabetes: A population-based cohort and sibling design study. Diabetes Care. 2015;**38**:2308-2315

[32] Clausen TD et al. Prelabor caesarean section and risk of childhood type 1 diabetes: A nationwide register-based cohort study. Epidemiology. 2016;**27**:547-555

[33] Samuelsson U et al. Caesarean section per se does not increase the risk of offspring developing type 1 diabetes: A Swedish population-based study. Diabetologia. 2015;**58**:2517-2524

[34] Cardwell CR et al. Maternal age at birth and childhood type 1 diabetes: A pooled analysis of 30 observational studies. Diabetes. 2010;**59**:486-494

[35] Chowdhury S. Puberty and type 1 diabetes. Indian. Journal of Endocrinology and Metabolism. 2015;**19**:51-54

[36] Kitabchi AE, Umpierrez GE, Murphy MB, Kreisberg RA. Hyperglycemic crises in adult patients with diabetes: A consensus statement from the American Diabetes Association. Diabetes Care. 2006;**29**(12):2739-2748. DOI: 10.2337/dc06-9916

[37] Misra S, Oliver NS. Diabetic ketoacidosis in adults. BMJ. 2015;**351**:h5660. DOI: 10.1136/bmj.h5660

[38] Maletkovic J, Drexler A. Diabetic ketoacidosis and hyperglycemic hyperosmolar state. Endocrinology and Metabolism Clinics of North America. 2013;**42**(4):677-695. DOI: 10.1016/j.ecl.2013.07.001

[39] Kitabchi AE, Umpierrez GE, Miles JM, Fisher JN. Hyperglycemic crises in adult patients with diabetes. Diabetes Care. 2009;**32**(7):1335-1343. DOI: 10.2337/dc09-9032

[40] Silverstein J, Klingensmith G, Copeland K, Plotnick L, Kaufman F, Laffel L, et al. Care of children and adolescents with type 1 diabetes: A statement of the American Diabetes Association. Diabetes Care. 2005;**28**(1):186-212. DOI: 10.2337/diacare.28.1.186

[41] Lindner LM, Rathmann W, Rosenbauer J. Inequalities in glycaemic control, hypoglycaemia and diabetic ketoacidosis according to socio-economic status and area-level deprivation in type 1 diabetes mellitus: A systematic review. Diabetic Medicine. 2018;**35**(1):12-32. DOI: 10.1111/dme.13519

[42] Joint British Diabetes Societies Inpatient Care Group. The Management of Diabetic Ketoacidosis in Adults. Association of British Clinical Diabetologists; 2021

[43] Bialo SR, Agrawal S, Boney CM, Quintos JB. Rare complications of pediatric diabetic ketoacidosis. World Journal of Diabetes. 2015;**6**(1):167-174. DOI: 10.4239/wjd.v6.i1.167

[44] Patel A, Singh D, Bhatt P, Thakkar B, Akingbola OA, Srivastav SK. Incidence, trends, and outcomes of cerebral Edema among children with diabetic ketoacidosis in the United States. Clinical Pediatrics. 2016;**55**(10):943-951. DOI: 10.1177/0009922815617975

[45] Brown TB. Cerebral oedema in childhood diabetic ketoacidosis: Is treatment a factor? Emergency Medicine Journal. 2004;**21**(2):141-144. DOI: 10.1136/emj.2002.001578

[46] Jameson J, Fauci AS, Kasper DL, Hauser SL, Longo DL, Loscalzo J, editors. Harrison's Principles of Internal Medicine. 20th ed. New York: McGraw-Hill Education; 2018

[47] DiMeglio LA, Evans-Molina C, Oram RA. Type 1 diabetes. Lancet. 2018;**391**(10138):2449-2462. DOI: 10.1016/S0140-6736(18)31320-5

[48] Vujosevic S, Aldington SJ, Silva P, Hernández C, Scanlon P, Peto T, et al. Screening for diabetic retinopathy: New perspectives and challenges. The Lancet Diabetes and Endocrinology. 2020;**8**(4):337-347. DOI: 10.1016/S2213-8587(19)30411-5. hdl:2434/881134

[49] Brownlee M, Aiello LP, Sun JK, Cooper ME, Feldman EL, Plutzky J, et al. Complications of Diabetes Mellitus. Williams Textbook of Endocrinology. Fourteenth Edition. Philadelphia: Elsevier; 2020. pp. 1438-1524

[50] Zimmet P, Alberti KGMM, Shaw J. Global and societal implications of the diabetes epidemic. Nature. 2001;**414**(6865):782-787. DOI: 10.1038/414782a

[51] Trivedi HS, Pang MMH, Campbell A, Saab P. Slowing the progression of chronic renal failure: Economic benefits and patients' perspectives. American Journal of Kidney Diseases. 2002;**39**(4):721-713. DOI: 10.1053/ajkd.2002.31990

[52] Mahapatra S, Firpo MT, Bacanamwo M. Inhibition of DNA methyltransferases and histone deacetylases induces bone marrow-derived multipotent adult progenitor cells to differentiate into endothelial cells. Ethnicity & Disease. 2010;**20**(1 Suppl. 1):S1-60-S1-64

[53] Huxley RR, Peters SA, Mishra GD, Woodward M. Risk of all-cause mortality and vascular events in women versus men with type 1 diabetes: A systematic review and meta-analysis. The Lancet. Diabetes and Endocrinology. 2015;**3**(3):198-206. DOI: 10.1016/S2213-8587(14)70248-7

[54] Sun J, Wang Y, Zhang X, Zhu S, He H. Prevalence of peripheral neuropathy in patients with diabetes: A systematic review and meta-analysis. Primary Care Diabetes. 2020;**14**(5):435-444

[55] Poulain C, Johanet C, Delcroix C, L'evy-Marchal C, Tubiana-Rufi N. Prevalence and clinical features of celiac disease in 950 children with type 1 diabetes in France. Diabetes & Metabolism. 2007;**33**(6):453-458

[56] Barera G, Bonfanti R, Viscardi M, et al. Occurrence of celiac disease after onset of type 1 diabetes: A 6-year prospective longitudinal study. Pediatrics. 2002;**109**(5):833-838

[57] Holmes GKT. Coeliac disease and type 1 diabetes mellitus—The case

for screening. Diabetic Medicine. 2001;**18**(3):169-177

[58] Ludvigsson JF, Ludvigsson J, Ekbom A, Montgomery SM. Celiac disease and risk of subsequent type 1 diabetes: A general population cohort study of children and adolescents. Diabetes Care. 2006;**29**(11):2483-2488

[59] Cerutti F, Bruno G, Chiarelli F, Lorini R, Meschi F, Sacchetti C. The diabetes study group of the italian society of pediatric endocrinology and diabetology. Younger age at onset and sex predict celiac disease in children and adolescents with type 1 diabetes. An Italian multicenter study. Diabetes Care. 2004;**27**(6):1294-1298

[60] Kakleas K, Kostaki M, Critselis E, et al. Gastric autoimmunity in children and adolescents with type 1 diabetes: A prospective study. Hormone Research in Pædiatrics. 2012;**77**(2):121-126

[61] De Block CEM, De Leeuw IH, Vertommen JJF, et al. Beta-cell, thyroid, gastric, adrenal and coeliac autoimmunity and HLA-DQ types in type 1 diabetes. Clinical and Experimental Immunology. 2001;**126**(2):236-241

[62] Fröhlich-Reiterer EE, Huber J, Katz H, et al. Do children and adolescents with type 1 diabetes mellitus have a higher frequency of parietal cell antibodies than healthy controls? Journal of Pediatric Gastroenterology and Nutrition. 2011;**52**(5):558-562

[63] Jaeger C, Hatziagelaki E, Petzoldt R, Bretzel RG. Comparative analysis of organ-specific autoantibodies and celiac disease-associated antibodies in type 1 diabetic patients, their first-degree relatives, and healthy control subjects. Diabetes Care. 2001;**24**(1):27-32

[64] Popoviciu MS, Kaka N, Sethi Y, Patel N, Chopra H, Cavalu S. Type 1 Diabetes Mellitus and Autoimmune Diseases: A Critical Review of the Association and the Application of Personalized Medicine. Journal of Personalized Medicine. 26 Feb 2023;**13**(3):422. DOI: 10.3390/jpm13030422

[65] Fichna M, Fichna P, Gryczy'nska M, Walkowiak J, Zurawek M, Sowi'nski J. Screening for associated autoimmune disorders in polish patients with Addison's disease. Endocrine. 2010;**37**(2):349-360

[66] Kakleas K, Soldatou A, Karachaliou F, Karavanaki K. Associated autoimmune diseases in children and adolescents with type 1 T1DM(T1DM). Autoimmunity Reviews. 2015;**14**(9):781-797

[67] Taïeb A, Picardo M. The definition and assessment of vitiligo: A consensus report of theVitiligo European task force. Pigment Cell Research Journal. 2007;**20**(1):27-35

[68] Kemp EH, Gavalas NG, Gawkrodger DJ, Weetman AP. Autoantibody responses to melanocytes in the depigmenting skin disease vitiligo. Autoimmunity Reviews. 2007;**6**(3):138-142

[69] Gopal KV, Rao GR, Kumar YR. Increased prevalence of thyroid dysfunction and T1DM in Indian vitiligo patients: A case-control study. Indian Dermatology Online Journal. 2014;**5**(4):456-460

[70] Shaikh SB, Haji IM, Doddamani P, Rahman M. Astudy of autoimmune polyglandular syndrome (PAS) in patients with type1 T1DM (T1DM) followed up at a teritiary care hospital. Journal of Clinical and Diagnostic Research. 2014;**8**(2):70-72

[71] Van Den Driessche A, Eenkhoorn V, Van Gaal L, De Block C. Type 1 diabetes

and autoimmune polyglandular syndrome: A clinical review. The Netherlands Journal of Medicine. 2009;**67**(11):376-387

[72] Ben-Skowronek I, Michalczyk A, Piekarski R, Wysocka Łukasik B, Banecka B. Type III polyglandular autoimmune syndromes in children with type 1 T1DM. Annals of Agricultural and Environmental Medicine. 2013;**20**(1):140-146

[73] Hermann G, Thon A, Mönkemöller K, et al. Comorbidity of type 1 diabetes and juvenile idiopathic arthritis. The Journal of Pediatrics. 2015;**166**(4):930-935.e3

Chapter 2

Prevalence and Incidence of Type 1 Diabetes in the World

Morteza Ghojazadeh, Majid Mobasseri, Fatemeh Pournaghi Azar and AliReza Lotfi

Abstract

Type 1 diabetes (T1D) is an autoimmune disease. The global prevalence of T1D is estimated to range from 0.8 to 4.6 per 1000 population. In most cases, the prevalence is higher, at 1–1.5 per 1000. In terms of incidence, variations have been noted based on geographical location, ethnicity, diagnostic criteria, birth season, age, and gender. Additionally, disease incidence exhibits differences across specific age groups and between sexes. The prevalence of this condition is higher among children than adults. The highest incidence occurs within the 10–14-year age group, followed by a gradual decline in prevalence as individuals age. In 2021, approximately 6% of adults reported receiving a physician's diagnosis of diabetes. It is notable that physician-diagnosed diabetes is more prevalent in men (7%) than in women (5%). Furthermore, it is clear that the prevalence of T1D increases with age. In adults under 35, it is 1%. In adults aged 75 and older, it is 16%. There is a growing incidence and prevalence of T1D worldwide. Insulin scarcity and its associated high costs will disproportionately affect underdeveloped and developing nations. Consequently, it becomes imperative for international organizations and individual countries to proactively implement preventive measures in response to these concerning trends.

Keywords: diabetes mellitus, incidence, prevalence, type 1, epidemiology

1. Introduction

The field of epidemiology is concerned with the study of the various factors that contribute to the incidence, prevalence, distribution, and process of disease. It also encompasses the investigation of strategies for the eradication or prevention of these factors [1]. In the context of type 1 diabetes (T1D), epidemiological research provides invaluable insights into the epidemiology of this disease, including data on its prevalence, incidence, and associated morbidity and mortality. This knowledge is essential for improving patient care, which is the ultimate objective of any medical activity. T1D mellitus is a chronic condition in which the pancreas produces little to no insulin [2]. Insulin is a hormone that regulates the level of glucose (sugar) in the blood [3]. Without enough insulin, the level of glucose in the blood will become too high. This type of diabetes is typically diagnosed in children and young adults, but it can occur at any age [4].

It is an autoimmune condition, whereby the body's immune system attacks and destroys the insulin-producing beta cells in the pancreas [5]. People with T1D require lifelong insulin therapy to survive [6, 7]. Management of the condition usually involves regular blood sugar monitoring [8], insulin injections or the use of an insulin pump [9], and careful management of diet [10] and exercise [11, 12]. T1D can lead to various complications if not properly managed, such as heart disease [13, 14], stroke [15], kidney disease [16], vision problems [17], and nerve damage [18]. However, with proper treatment and management, people with T1D can lead full and healthy lives.

There is no doubt that the incidence of T1D is on the rise worldwide. This autoimmune condition, where the body's immune system attacks and destroys insulin-producing cells in the pancreas, is a growing concern [19]. Historically, T1D was most commonly diagnosed in children and adolescents, hence its former name "juvenile diabetes" [20]. However, it can occur at any age [21]. In recent decades, there has been a noticeable rise in the incidence of T1D, especially in developed countries [22]. While the exact reasons for this increase are not fully understood, it is clear that a combination of genetic predisposition and environmental factors is responsible [23].

Several studies have suggested that factors such as changes in diet, lower levels of physical activity [24], as well as early childhood exposure to certain viruses [25] may play a role in the increasing incidence of T1D. Additionally, there is ongoing research into the potential impact of factors like climate change [26], pollution, and changes in the gut microbiome [27].

Efforts to understand and address the increasing incidence of T1D are ongoing, with a focus on genetics, immunology, and environmental factors. Additionally, advances in treatments and therapies, including technologies for glucose monitoring and insulin delivery, aim to improve the management of T1D for those who are affected by it [9]. The incidence of T1D varies across different populations, and it is often presented as the number of new cases per 100,000 people per year. In many Western countries, the incidence is increasing, particularly among children. The rise in incidence is a cause for concern, and researchers and healthcare providers are actively studying the factors contributing to this trend.

A diagnosis of T1D is typically made on the basis of blood sugar test results and the presence of a constellation of symptoms [28]. The most common symptoms of T1D are as follows:

- Abnormal thirst and dry mouth
- Sudden weight loss
- Frequent urination
- Lack of energy, tiredness
- Constant hunger
- Blurred vision
- Bedwetting

It can be challenging to diagnose T1D, and additional tests may be necessary to confirm a diagnosis.

2. Incidence of T1D

The prevalence and incidence of T1D are different because they measure different aspects of the disease within a population. The term prevalence is used to describe the total number of cases of a disease in a given population at a specific point in time. It represents the proportion of individuals in a population who have the disease at that time. On the other hand, incidence measures the rate of new cases of a disease that develop within a specific time period. It represents the risk of developing the disease over a certain period, often expressed as the number of new cases per unit of population at risk.

The prevalence of T1D can be influenced by factors such as the longevity of individuals with the condition, as well as changes in disease management and treatment that can affect the overall number of people living with the disease at a certain point in time. The incidence of T1D, on the other hand, reflects the rate at which new cases are diagnosed within a given population. This can be influenced by factors such as genetic predisposition, environmental triggers, and changes in diagnostic criteria or detection methods. In summary, the prevalence of T1D reflects the total number of existing cases at a specific point in time, while the incidence measures the rate of new cases developing over time.

In 2017, there were 9 million individuals diagnosed with T1D [29]. The majority of these individuals reside in high-income countries (**Figure 1**). Despite extensive research, the underlying cause of this disease and the means to prevent it remain unknown.

In accordance with the projections set forth by the World Health Organization (WHO), diabetes is expected to become the fifth leading cause of mortality on a global scale by the year 2030. T1D, also known as juvenile diabetes or insulin-dependent diabetes, represents the second most prevalent form of diabetes, accounting for approximately 5–10% of all diagnosed cases [31]. It has been reported that there are over 65,000 new cases of T1D in children worldwide each year, with the incidence rate increasing by approximately 3% annually [32].

Epidemiological studies have indicated that the incidence and prevalence of T1D have increased significantly in recent years, with a particularly marked increase

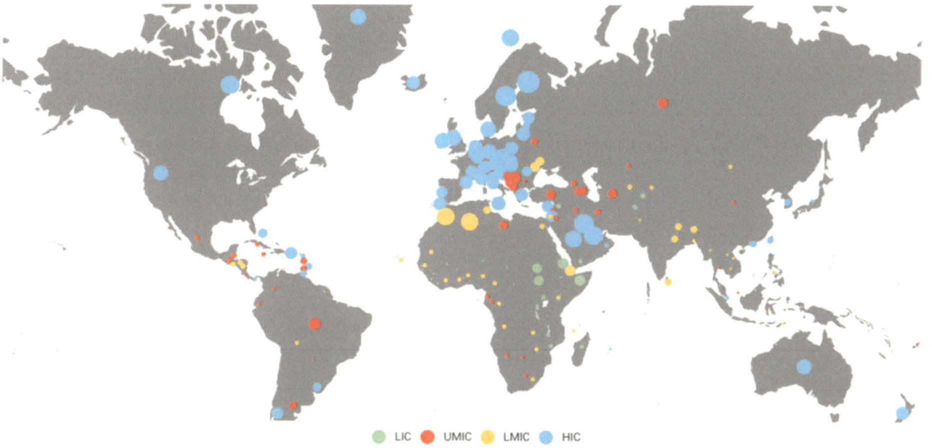

Figure 1.
*Geographical distribution map showing the incidence of type 1 diabetes in 2021 [30]. * HIC=High-income country; LMIC = Lower-middle income country; LIC = Low-income country; and UMIC=Upper-middle income country.*

Year	Prevalence		Incidence		Mortality		DALYs	
1990–1999	0.49 (0.46–0.52)	<0.001	0.88 (0.86–0.91)	<0.001	0.69 (0.56–0.82)	<0.001	0.66 (0.56–0.76)	<0.001
2000–2009	0.96 (0.94–0.97)	<0.001	1.41 (1.32–1.50)	<0.001	−1.46 (−1.99 to −0.93)	<0.001	−0.86 (−1.25 to −0.47)	<0.001
2010–2019	1.09 (1.04–1.14)	<0.001	1.35 (1.27–1.44)	<0.001	−0.48 (−0.69 to −0.29)	<0.001	−0.03 (−0.20 to 0.14)	0.70
1990–2019	0.85 (0.82–0.87)	<0.001	1.22 (1.18–1.27)	<0.001	−0.41 (−0.6 to −0.22)	<0.001	−0.07 (−0.21 to 0.07)	0.32

**AAPC average annual percentage change.*

Table 1.
Global AAPCs in prevalence, incidence, mortality, and DALYs of type 1 diabetes among adolescents and young adults aged 10–24 years [39].

observed in children under the age of five [33]. Diabetes mellitus (DM), which has been designated the inaugural non-infectious epidemic of the modern era, has a multitude of long-term health consequences that impact patients' well-being and place a significant burden on the healthcare system. The disease results in a multitude of disabilities and a considerable mortality rate, largely attributable to its numerous chronic vascular complications.

The International Diabetes Federation (IDF) estimates that there are currently 537 million people with diabetes worldwide [34]. This figure is projected to reach 783 million by 2045 [35]. T1D accounts for 15–20% of all cases and is particularly prevalent in European populations.

The rising incidence of T1D in adolescents and young adults represents a significant challenge for global healthcare systems. The incidence of T1D in children and adolescents is rising at a consistent rate, with the current incidence estimated at 22.9 new cases per year per 100,000 children up to the age of 15 years in Germany [36]. The rising incidence of T1D has been attributed to rapid economic development and urbanization. The financial burden of diabetes care is at least 3.2 times greater than the average per capita healthcare expenditure, rising to 9.4 times in the presence of complications [37]. A multicenter study in the United States demonstrated that the overall unadjusted estimated incidence rates of T1D in youths increased by 1.4% annually from 2002 to 2012 [38]. Therefore, it is crucial to comprehend the global burden of T1D in adolescents in order to optimize the utilization of healthcare resources in different countries (**Table 1**).

In 2021, the estimated global prevalence of individuals living with T1D was approximately 8.4 million, with 500,000 new cases diagnosed that year. It is projected that by 2040, the number of individuals living with T1D will reach 13.5–17.4 million [22]. The life expectancy of a 10-year-old child diagnosed with T1D is, on average, 13 years in low-income countries and 65 years in high-income countries. Significant complications, including cardiac diastolic dysfunction, dyslipidemia and albuminuria, have been documented in adolescents with T1D, with evidence of endothelial dysfunction emerging even earlier during childhood. Moreover, approximately 30% of patients with T1D develop end-stage kidney disease over the course of their lifetime [40]. Furthermore, T1D is associated with a poor quality of life and psychological burden [41]. It is therefore becoming increasingly evident that the rise in the incidence of T1D worldwide represents a significant challenge to public health. The prevalence of T1D is increasing at an annual rate of 0.34% [22]. The role of environmental factors in the onset of the autoimmune process that leads to the destruction of β-cells has been the subject of extensive research. Furthermore, perinatal parameters, such as mode of delivery and maternal and childhood diet, and ecological contributors, such as atmospheric pollution and climatic conditions, have been proposed as potential correlates of the incidence of T1D. The increasing prevalence of obesity, which results in insulin resistance and dyslipidemia, has been hypothesized to accelerate the onset of T1D in genetically susceptible individuals. Understanding the epidemiology of T1D is crucial for developing effective public health strategies. It is important to consider geographic, gender, age, seasonal, and ethnic factors when studying the prevalence and incidence of the disease. These insights can inform future research and healthcare initiatives.

Estimating the epidemiology of T1D involves analyzing incidence, prevalence, and risk factors for the disease. The availability of accurate data on the prevalence, incidence, associated mortality and life expectancy of T1D is essential for informing public health policy. However, such data are currently scarce. The incidence of T1D varies globally, with higher rates in countries further from the equator. Scandinavia has some of the highest rates, with approximately 25 new cases per 100,000 individuals each year, while rates in other regions may be lower. The prevalence of T1D is increasing worldwide, particularly in younger age groups. It is estimated that the global prevalence of T1D is increasing by approximately 3% annually, although regional variations exist. The incidence rate of T1D has increased 3–4% annually in European countries from 1989 to 2013, indicating a doubling incidence rate over 20 years (**Figure 2**) [42].

Furthermore, an increasing annual rate of 1.8% in the United States (2002–2012) and 2.8% worldwide (1990–1999) for T1D has been documented. In 2019, the International Diabetes Federation (IDF) estimated the highest number of T1D patients (aged 0–19 years) in Europe, at 296.5 per 1000 individuals [35]. South and East Asia, and the Middle East and North Africa (MENA) regions were the third and fourth most affected regions globally, respectively. In 2021, the International Diabetes Federation (IDF) reported that the number of individuals with T1D aged 0–19 years in Iran was 8.2 per 1000 people [35].

Several factors can influence the incidence of T1D (**Figure 3**). Here are some of the key factors:

Genetics: T1D has a significant genetic component. Those with a family history of the condition are at an elevated risk of developing it. Genetics plays a pivotal role in the pathogenesis of T1D [43]. People with a family history of the condition have a higher risk of developing T1D. The risk is higher if a parent or sibling has the condition. Specific genes, such as those in the human leukocyte antigen (HLA) complex, have been identified as being associated with an increased risk of T1D [44]. However, having these genes does not guarantee that a person will develop the condition, as environmental factors also seem to play a role. Environmental triggers, such as certain viruses, may interact with genetic predisposition to initiate the autoimmune process that leads to the development of T1D [45].

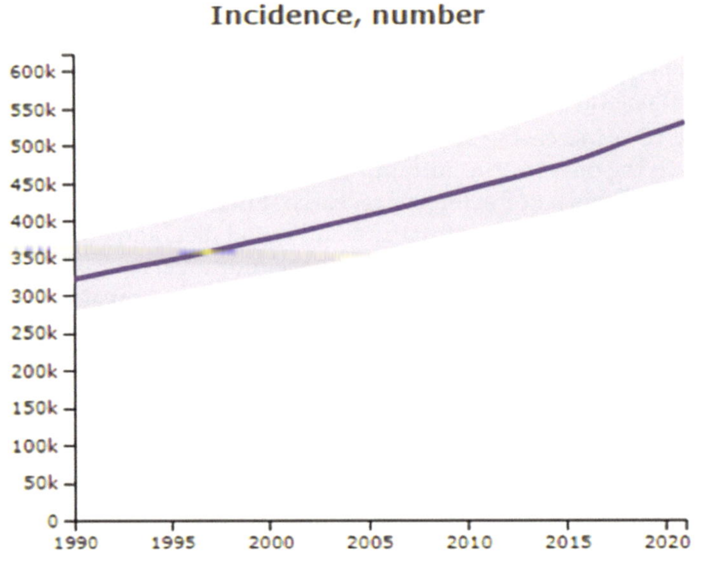

Figure 2.
Global incidence of death due to T1D in both sexes and all age groups.

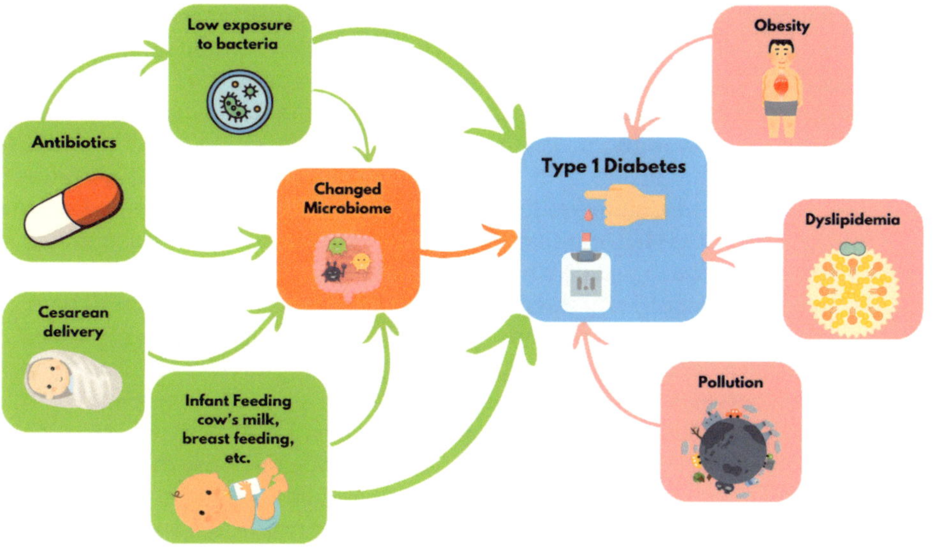

Figure 3.
Risk factors contributing to the rise in T1D incidence.

The development of T1D is influenced by a combination of genetic and environmental factors. Several genes have been identified to play a role in the predisposition to T1D. Some of these genes include:

1. HLA complex: Variations in the human leukocyte antigen (HLA) genes, particularly the HLA-DQA1, HLA-DQB1, and HLA-DRB1, have been strongly linked to an increased risk of T1D [46, 47].

2. INS gene: Variants in the insulin (INS) gene have been associated with an increased risk of developing T1D [48, 49].

3. CTLA-4 gene: The cytotoxic T-lymphocyte-associated Antigen 4 (CTLA-4) gene is another gene that has been implicated in the genetic susceptibility to T1D [50].

4. PTPN22 gene: Variations in the protein tyrosine phosphatase, non-receptor type 22 (PTPN22) gene have also been linked to an elevated risk of T1D [51, 52].

These are just a few examples of the many genes that have been found to have associations with T1D. However, it is important to note that having these genetic variants does not necessarily mean a person will develop T1D, as environmental factors also play a significant role in the onset of the disease.

Autoimmune factors: T1D is an autoimmune disease, meaning the body's immune system mistakenly targets and destroys insulin-producing beta cells in the pancreas. Environmental factors such as viral infections, exposure to certain toxins, and early childhood diet may trigger this autoimmune response in genetically susceptible individuals. Autoimmune factors play a significant role in the occurrence of T1D. In T1D, the body's immune system mistakenly attacks and destroys the insulin-producing beta cells in the pancreas. This autoimmune response leads to a lack of insulin, which is essential for regulating blood sugar levels. The exact trigger for this autoimmune response is not known, but genetic predisposition and environmental factors, such as viral infections, are believed to play a role. Environmental factors, including viral infections and early exposure to certain foods or cow's milk, may also trigger the autoimmune response in individuals with a genetic predisposition [53].

Overall, the autoimmune factors in T1D lead to the destruction of insulin-producing cells, resulting in a lack of insulin production and an inability to regulate blood sugar levels. This understanding has led to research into potential treatments aimed at modulating the autoimmune response to preserve beta cell function in individuals with T1D.

Viral infections: Certain viral infections, particularly in early childhood, have been linked to an increased risk of developing T1D. Viruses such as enteroviruses and rotaviruses have been studied in relation to the development of the condition. The relationship between viral infections and T1D is an area of active research. Some studies suggest that certain viral infections, particularly enteroviruses such as coxsackievirus and rotavirus, may trigger an autoimmune response that leads to the development of T1D in genetically susceptible individuals [54, 55]. In these cases, the viral infection is thought to set off a chain of events that result in the immune system mistakenly attacking the insulin-producing cells in the pancreas.

However, it is important to note that the exact role of viral infections in the development of T1D is complex and not fully understood. Not everyone who experiences these infections develops diabetes, and many individuals diagnosed with T1D do not have a history of viral infections preceding their diagnosis. Research in this area is ongoing, and scientists continue to investigate the potential links between viral infections and the development of T1D. Understanding these relationships can potentially lead to new preventive and treatment strategies.

The hygiene hypothesis posits that exposure to microbes during childhood facilitates the maturation and development of the immune system. Consequently, the absence of such exposure is associated with an elevated risk of autoimmune diseases [56, 57]. The hypothesis is supported by a significant negative correlation between the incidence of T1D by country and mortality from parasitic and infectious diseases, tuberculosis, respiratory infections and diarrheal diseases. In addition to serving as an indicator of the quality of healthcare provided, infectious disease mortality also serves as an indicator of the overall infectious burden [58]. Moreover, maternal infections during pregnancy have been linked to a reduced risk of developing T1D [59]. It is important to note, however, that reverse causality may be a factor in the observed association between T1D and infectious diseases. This implies that the lower incidence of T1D in low-income countries may be related to lower survival rates of children due to the provision of poor-quality health services. Another factor that is associated with an increased risk of developing T1D is exposure to antibiotics [60]. It has been demonstrated that exposure to a single antibiotic during the first year of life does not increase the probability of developing T1D. Nevertheless, exposure to two or more antibiotic treatments during the first year of life has been identified as a significant predictive factor for the subsequent development of T1D [61].

Early childhood diet: Some research suggests that the timing of introduction to certain foods, such as cow's milk and cereals, during infancy may influence the risk of developing T1D [62]. Research suggests that childhood diet may play a role in the development of T1D. Studies have explored the potential link between early diet and the risk of developing T1D, with some evidence pointing to factors such as the timing of introduction to certain foods, breastfeeding, and the consumption of cow's milk and gluten [63, 64]. However, the precise relationship between childhood diet and T1D is complex and continues to be an area of active research. While diet is not the sole factor in the development of T1D, it is considered to be one of the potential environmental influences alongside genetic predisposition. Additionally, factors such as geography, with higher incidence rates observed in certain regions, as well as other environmental influences, may also play a role in the development of T1D.

The incidence of T1D has been observed to vary geographically, with higher rates generally reported in countries further from the equator. This suggests a potential correlation between geographical location and the risk of developing T1D. Some studies have linked lower levels of sunlight exposure and vitamin D deficiency in regions further from the equator to an increased risk of developing T1D [65]. There is evidence to suggest that incidence rates of T1D vary with geographical location and climate, with higher rates observed in northern countries (**Figure 4**) [66].

Exposure to elevated concentrations of ozone in the atmosphere, both postnatally and during gestation, is associated with an elevated risk of developing T1D [67]. The diabetogenic effects of ozone are thought to be exerted by increasing oxidative stress [68, 69], inflammation [70], and apoptosis [71]. Furthermore, in animal studies, ozone has been demonstrated to induce insulin resistance [72]. It is now well-established that exposure to particulate matter of 10 μm (PM10) and 2.5 μm (PM2.5) in diameter in children before the age of 5 years is an important prognostic factor for the development of T1D. Inhalation of particulate matter of this size can result in a number of adverse health effects. Furthermore, evidence indicates that it can also promote inflammation [73] and stimulate the release of interleukin 1β (IL-1β), which plays a pivotal role in the destruction of β-cells in T1D [74]. Other air pollutants with a strong correlation with the incidence of T1D include nitrogen oxides, which encompass both nitrogen oxide (NO) and nitrogen dioxide (NO_2). A well-established dose-dependent association has been observed between increased ambient levels of nitrogen oxides and IL6. In addition to the aforementioned pollutants, numerous other environmental contaminants, the concentrations of which are elevated due to human activity, have been demonstrated to increase the risk of developing T1D in animal models. Nevertheless, there is a paucity of human studies in this field. Such contaminants include bisphenol A, organochlorine pollutants, mercury, and aluminum [75–79].

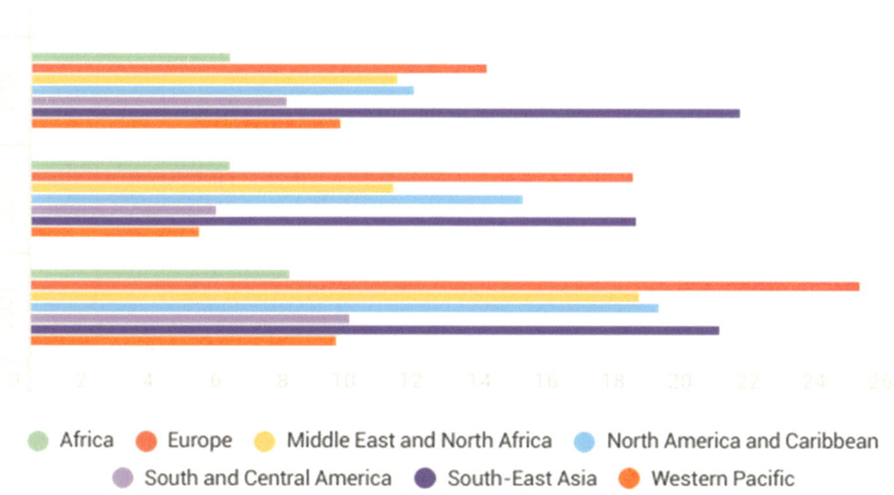

Figure 4.
Incidence of T1D in children aged 0–14 years across different continents, per 1000 individuals.

Research suggests that there may be a gender-based difference in the occurrence of T1D [80]. Historically, T1D has been more prevalent in males than in females [81, 82]. However, more recent studies indicate that the incidence of T1D is increasing at a faster rate in females than in males. This means that the gender gap is narrowing.

It is important to note that the reasons behind these gender differences are not entirely clear and may be influenced by various genetic, hormonal, and environmental factors. Research in this area is ongoing to better understand the relationship between gender and the occurrence of T1D.

Age can have an impact on the occurrence of T1D. T1D is most commonly diagnosed in children and young adults, although it can occur at any age. It was traditionally known as "juvenile diabetes" because of its frequent onset in children. However, it is important to note that adults can also develop T1D.

In general, the risk of developing T1D decreases with age [83], but it is not exclusive to any particular age group. While children and young adults make up a significant portion of those diagnosed with T1D, cases can also occur in older individuals.

Seasonal differences can have some impact on the incidence of T1D, although the exact reasons are not fully understood. Some studies suggest that there might be a slightly higher incidence of T1D in winter months or colder climates [84], while others have found different patterns [85].

The incidence of T1D varies across different ethnic groups [86, 87]. For example, individuals of European descent have a higher risk of developing T1D compared to individuals of other ethnic backgrounds. In contrast, populations of African, Hispanic, and Asian descent generally have a lower incidence of T1D. It is important to note that these observations are based on general trends and may not apply universally to all individuals within a particular ethnic group. Additionally, ongoing research is furthering our understanding of the complex interplay between genetics, environment, and lifestyle factors in the development of T1D.

It is clear that a number of factors that have become increasingly prevalent in recent decades are contributing to the rising incidence of T1D. There is no doubt that modulation of the microbiome represents a pivotal mechanism through which numerous environmental factors, including breastfeeding, mode of delivery, childhood diet, antibiotic use, and lack of microbial exposure, exert their influence on the risk of T1D.

3. Prevalence of T1D

The prevalence of T1D has been increasing worldwide, particularly among children. According to the International Diabetes Federation (IDF), approximately 1.1 million children and adolescents under the age of 20 were estimated to have T1D globally, with around 128,900 new cases diagnosed each year [88]. The global prevalence of T1D is estimated to range from 0.8 to 4.6 per 1000 population, with a higher incidence of 1–1.5 per 1000 in most cases [89]. With regard to its incidence, discrepancies have been observed across countries, races, diagnoses, birth seasons, age groups, and sexes (**Figure 5**).

In 2021, the global prevalence of T1D was estimated to be 8.4 million cases (95% uncertainty interval 8.1–8.8) [19]. Of the total number of individuals, 1.5 million (18%) were younger than 20 years of age, 5.4 million (64%) were aged between 20 and 59 years, and 1.6 million (19%) were aged 60 years or older. In that year, 0.5 million new cases were diagnosed (with a median age of onset of 29 years), and approximately 35,000 individuals who were not diagnosed died within 12 months

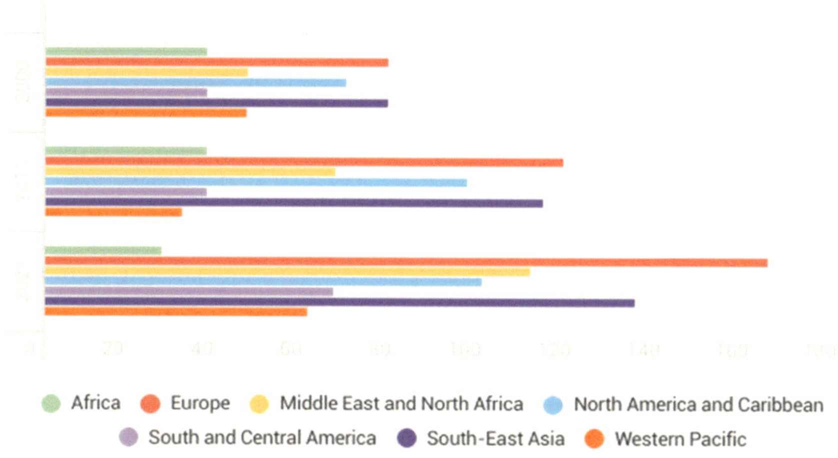

Figure 5.
Prevalence of T1D in children aged 0-14 years across different continents, per 1000 individuals.

of the onset of symptoms. One in five individuals with T1D resided in low-income and lower-middle-income countries. The remaining life expectancy of a 10-year-old diagnosed with T1D in 2021 ranged from a mean of 13 years in low-income countries to 65 years in high-income countries. It was estimated that 3.7 million prevalent cases were missing in 2021. By 2040, it is anticipated that there will be an increase in prevalent cases to 13.5–17.4 million (60–107% higher than in 2021), with the greatest relative increase in low-income and lower-middle-income countries (**Figure 6**).

In terms of regional prevalence:

- Scandinavia has one of the highest rates of T1D in the world [90].
- Finland has one of the highest rates of T1D in the world with nearly 60 in every 100,000 people affected.

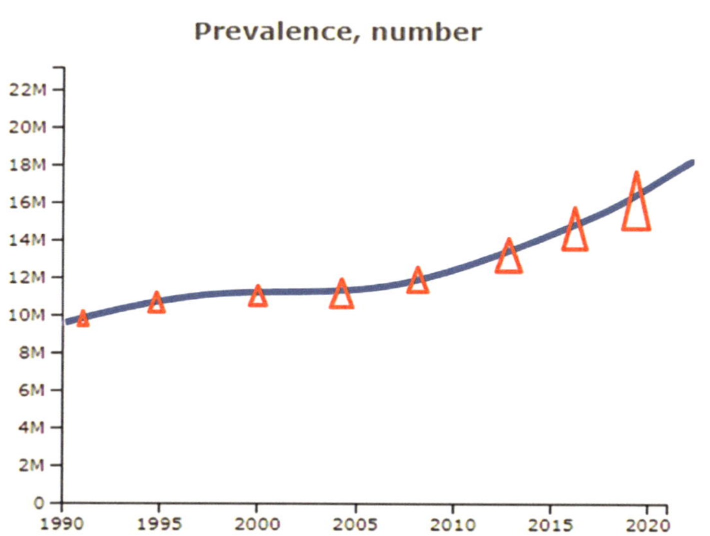

Figure 6.
Type 1 diabetes prevalence trends (1990–2020).

- In the United States, around 1.25 million individuals have T1D [91].

The prevalence of T1D varies around the world. Here are some estimates for the prevalence of T1D in different countries based on data available up to September 2021:

- Finland: Finland has one of the highest rates of T1D in the world, with around 65 in 100,000 children being diagnosed annually [92].

- Sweden: Sweden also has a relatively high prevalence of T1D, with around 43 in 100,000 children being diagnosed annually [93].

- United States: In the US, the estimated prevalence is around 2.15 per 1000 individuals under the age of 19 [94].

- United Kingdom: The reported prevalence rate of T1D in England and Wales was 204.5 per 100,000 population in the United Kingdom [95].

- Germany: In 2020, the prevalence of T1D in Germany was estimated to be 235.5 per 100,000 persons [96].

- -India: The prevalence of T1D in India is lower compared to Western countries, with an estimated annual incidence of about 3.2 per 100,000 population.

Canada has a similar prevalence to the USA, with approximately 1 in 600 children affected [97].

In China, the prevalence of T1D is much lower, with an estimated 1 in 10,000 children affected.

Generally, developed countries in North America and Europe tend to have higher rates of T1D compared to developing countries in Asia, Africa, and South America. The International Diabetes Federation (IDF) estimated that approximately 98,200 children develop T1D each year, with a global prevalence of around 1 in 500 among children and adolescents.

Epidemiological research on T1D has historically concentrated on the pediatric age group. However, recent data in adults has corroborated the assertion that T1D is a disease of all ages, manifesting with a broad clinical spectrum. The prevalence of T1D shows no significant sex-related differences, meaning it affects both males and females similarly. However, it does show an overall increasing trend, which is a cause for concern. Researchers and healthcare professionals are continuously working to understand and address the factors contributing to this increase. The estimated global prevalence of T1D among children aged 0–14 years was approximately 0.4%. This can vary by country and region, but this statistic provides a general approximation.

The life expectancy of T1D patients has been improving over the years, thanks to advancements in medical treatments and technology [98]. With proper management of the condition, including regular blood sugar monitoring, insulin therapy, and a healthy lifestyle, many individuals with T1D can live long and the objective is to facilitate the fulfillment of lives. It is, however, of the utmost importance that individuals with T1D work in close collaboration with healthcare professionals in order to effectively manage their condition. A number of factors, including overall health, access to healthcare and lifestyle choices, can all impact life expectancy. Awareness of the incidence and prevalence rates of T1D and its complications enables the planning

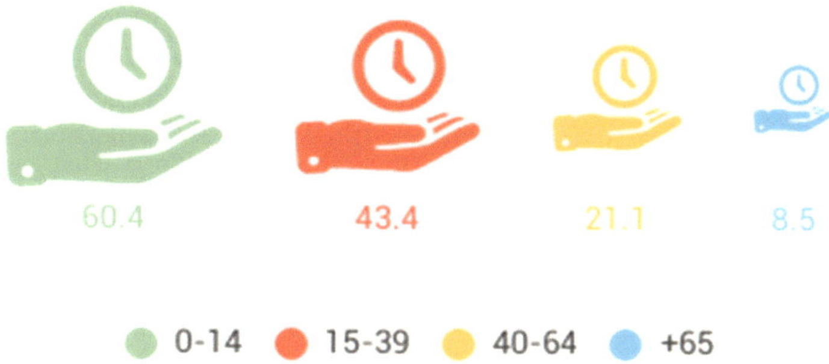

Figure 7.
Maximum mean remaining life-years by age group at onset [29].

and management of the human and financial resources available in areas where they are most needed, allowing for the optimal allocation of resources to meet the needs of affected individuals. Moreover, it allows for the assessment of the efficacy of preventive measures. It is therefore evident that such data are indispensable for the effective management and planning of healthcare services. In the initial period following a diagnosis of T1D, resources are allocated to outpatient care, pharmaceuticals, and self-monitoring. No chronic complications have been observed. It is only in the context of acute complications, which are relatively inexpensive unless they necessitate hospital admission, that costs may be incurred. Despite the preventive information campaigns that have been conducted, a considerable proportion of patients with T1D continue to present with ketoacidosis at the time of diagnosis [99]. Subsequently, costs are doubled due to the necessity of inpatient treatment for chronic complications. The mean cost per patient with T1D in the first year after diagnosis is approximately 3000 euros [89]. In the event that no chronic complications arise during the follow-up period, the cost is estimated to be approximately 1300 euros per individual per year. In patients with chronic complications, hospital admissions and social expenses may result in an overall mean cost of 3300 euros per patient per year. The global prevalence of T1D is considerable, with an anticipated increase in incidence, particularly in countries with limited resources. The majority of new cases and those already present are in adults. The considerable discrepancy in reported prevalence rates highlights the premature mortality associated with T1D and presents a crucial opportunity to enhance the lives of individuals with this condition (**Figure** 7).

4. Conclusions

Despite the peak incidence of T1D occurring during early adolescence, there has been a notable increase in the diagnosis of T1D in adulthood compared to childhood. This is attributed to the growing recognition of adult-onset T1D and the extended lifespan of adults. The geographical variations in incidence remain consistent, with the highest prevalence observed in Northern Europe and the lowest in Asia. The onset of T1D in adulthood is typically less acute than in childhood and confers a lower, though still considerable, risk of complications and early mortality. New interventions to delay the onset of T1D are being developed, and screening for individuals at risk at birth is becoming increasingly available. By elucidating the precise mechanisms through which environmental factors contribute to the pathogenesis of T1D, we can gain insight into the complex etiology of the disease, identify novel risk factors that remain undiscovered, and ultimately determine the public health measures necessary to prevent the increase in new T1D cases. The most evident yet formidable measures to address the surge in T1D cases are to promote a healthy lifestyle and diet, advocate for cesarean section alternatives and antibiotic prescriptions only when medically necessary, encourage breastfeeding and curtail environmental pollution.

The effects of a lack of insulin are more pronounced in children than in adults, and children are at a greater risk of developing diabetic ketoacidosis at a faster rate. Prior studies have indicated that there are geographic differences in the trends of T1D. A cross-sectional multicenter study of 3.47 million youths (aged 19 years or younger) in the USA revealed a significant increase in the estimated prevalence of T1D, from 1.48 cases per 1000 youths to 2.15 cases per 1000 youths [94]. The 10th edition of the International Diabetes Federation Atlas reports that the incidence of T1D in children and adolescents varies considerably across different countries and is increasing in many of them. A significant number of countries, particularly those with a low or middle social development index (SDI), are lacking in high-quality data regarding trends in T1D in adolescents. It is therefore imperative to gain a deeper understanding of the T1D burden in adolescents and to provide local governments with more detailed information in order to facilitate the management of this burden.

The prevalence of T1D among adolescents and young adults is a growing global health concern, particularly in countries with less well-developed economies. The global burden of T1D among adolescents is substantial, although there has been a decline in mortality and DALY rates over the past three decades due to advances in healthcare. Given the ongoing increase in the incidence and severity of T1D among adolescents and young adults, there is an urgent need for the implementation of lifestyle modification programmed in childhood.

In 2022, approximately 8.75 million individuals with diabetes were living with the condition, with 1.52 million of those being under the age of 20 [34]. The precise etiology of T1D remains elusive. Nevertheless, research indicates that the likelihood of developing the condition is marginally elevated in the event that a family member is afflicted with it. Additionally, environmental factors, such as exposure to a viral infection, have been identified as potential triggers for an autoimmune reaction that may lead to the development of T1D. At this time, there is no known method of preventing T1D, nor is there a cure for the condition.

Acknowledgements

The authors would like to acknowledge the Endocrine Research Center, Tabriz University of Medical Sciences, Tabriz, Iran and Research Center for Evidence-based Medicine, Iranian EBM Centre: A JBI Centre of Excellence, Faculty of Medicine, Tabriz University of Medical Sciences, Tabriz, Iran.

Conflict of interest

The authors declare no conflict of interest.

Author details

Morteza Ghojazadeh[1], Majid Mobasseri[2], Fatemeh Pournaghi Azar[1]
and AliReza Lotfi[3]*

1 Research Center for Evidence-based Medicine, Iranian EBM Centre: A JBI Centre of Excellence, Faculty of Medicine, Tabriz University of Medical Sciences, Tabriz, Iran

2 Endocrine Research Center, Tabriz University of Medical Sciences, Tabriz, Iran

3 Student Research Committee, Tabriz University of Medical Sciences, Tabriz, Iran

*Address all correspondence to: lotfialireza2003@gmail.com

References

[1] Evans AS. Epidemiological concepts. Bacterial Infections of Humans: Epidemiology and Control. 2009:1-50. DOI: 10.1007/978-0-387-09843-2_1

[2] Syed FZ. Type 1 diabetes mellitus. Annals of Internal Medicine. 2022;**175**(3):Itc33-itc48

[3] Rahman MS, Hossain KS, Das S, Kundu S, Adegoke EO, Rahman MA, et al. Role of insulin in health and disease: An update. International Journal of Molecular Sciences. 2021;**22**(12). DOI: 10.3390%2Fijms22126403

[4] Vanderniet JA, Jenkins AJ, Donaghue KC. Epidemiology of type 1 diabetes. Current Cardiology Reports. 2022;**24**(10):1455-1465

[5] Gillespie KM. Type 1 diabetes: Pathogenesis and prevention. CMAJ. 2006;**175**(2):165-170

[6] Powers AC. Type 1 diabetes mellitus: Much progress, many opportunities. The Journal of Clinical Investigation. 2021;**131**(8). DOI: 10.1172/jci142242

[7] Lucier J, Weinstock RS, Doerr C. Type 1 Diabetes (Nursing). In: StatPearls. Treasure Island (FL): StatPearls Publishing; 2024

[8] Smith A, Harris C. Type 1 diabetes: Management strategies. American Family Physician. 2018;**98**(3):154-162

[9] Beck RW, Bergenstal RM, Laffel LM, Pickup JC. Advances in technology for management of type 1 diabetes. Lancet. 2019;**394**(10205):1265-1273

[10] Gardemann C, Knowles S, Marquardt T. Managing type 1 diabetes mellitus with a ketogenic diet. Endocrinology, Diabetes & Metabolism Case Reports. 2023;**2023**(3). DOI: 10.1530/edm-23-0008

[11] Riddell MC, Gallen IW, Smart CE, Taplin CE, Adolfsson P, Lumb AN, et al. Exercise management in type 1 diabetes: A consensus statement. The Lancet Diabetes and Endocrinology. 2017;**5**(5):377-390

[12] Colberg SR. Nutrition and exercise performance in adults with type 1 diabetes. Canadian Journal of Diabetes. 2020;**44**(8):750-758

[13] Haji M, Erqou S, Fonarow GC, Echouffo-Tcheugui JB. Type 1 diabetes and risk of heart failure: A systematic review and meta-analysis. Diabetes Research and Clinical Practice. 2023;**202**:110805

[14] Liu Z, Wang H, Yang Z, Lu Y, Zou C. Causal associations between type 1 diabetes mellitus and cardiovascular diseases: A Mendelian randomization study. Cardiovascular Diabetology. 2023;**22**(1):236

[15] Zou X, Zhang L, Wang L, Wang S, Zeng Y. Exploring the causality of type 1 diabetes and stroke risk: A Mendelian randomization study and meta-analysis. Molecular Neurobiology. 2023;**60**(12):6814-6825

[16] Rivetti G, Hursh BE, Miraglia Del Giudice E, Marzuillo P. Acute and chronic kidney complications in children with type 1 diabetes mellitus. Pediatric Nephrology. 2023;**38**(5):1449-1458

[17] Bailes BK. Diabetes mellitus and its chronic complications. AORN Journal. 2002;**76**(2) 266-76, 78-82; quiz 83-6. DOI: 10.1016/s0001-2092(06)61065-x

[18] Galiero R, Caturano A, Vetrano E, Beccia D, Brin C, Alfano M, et al. Peripheral neuropathy in diabetes mellitus: Pathogenetic mechanisms and diagnostic options. International Journal of Molecular Sciences. 2023;**24**(4). DOI: 10.3390/ijms24043554

[19] Gregory GA, Robinson TIG, Linklater SE, Wang F, Colagiuri S, de Beaufort C, et al. Global incidence, prevalence, and mortality of type 1 diabetes in 2021 with projection to 2040: A modelling study. The Lancet Diabetes and Endocrinology. 2022;**10**(10):741-760

[20] Maahs DM, West NA, Lawrence JM, Mayer-Davis EJ. Epidemiology of type 1 diabetes. Endocrinology and Metabolism Clinics of North America. 2010;**39**(3):481-497

[21] Lucier J, Weinstock RS. Type 1 diabetes. In: StatPearls. Treasure Island (FL): StatPearls Publishing; 2024

[22] Ogrotis I, Koufakis T, Kotsa K. Changes in the global epidemiology of type 1 diabetes in an evolving landscape of environmental factors: Causes, challenges, and opportunities. Medicina (Kaunas, Lithuania). 2023;**59**(4). DOI: 10.3390%2Fmedicina59040668

[23] Esposito S, Toni G, Tascini G, Santi E, Berioli MG, Principi N. Environmental factors associated with type 1 diabetes. Frontiers in Endocrinology (Lausanne). 2019;**10**:592

[24] Czenczek-Lewandowska E, Leszczak J, Baran J, Weres A, Wyszyńska J, Lewandowski B, et al. Levels of physical activity in children and adolescents with type 1 diabetes in relation to the healthy comparators and to the method of insulin therapy used. International Journal of Environmental Research and Public Health. 2019;**16**(18). DOI: 10.3390/ijerph16183498

[25] Principi N, Berioli MG, Bianchini S, Esposito S. Type 1 diabetes and viral infections: What is the relationship? Journal of Clinical Virology. 2017;**96**:26-31

[26] Ratter-Rieck JM, Roden M, Herder C. Diabetes and climate change: Current evidence and implications for people with diabetes, clinicians and policy stakeholders. Diabetologia. 2023;**66**(6):1003-1015

[27] Zhou H, Sun L, Zhang S, Zhao X, Gang X, Wang G. Evaluating the causal role of gut microbiota in type 1 diabetes and its possible pathogenic mechanisms. Frontiers in Endocrinology. 2020;**11**. DOI: 10.3389/fendo.2020.00125

[28] DiMeglio LA, Evans-Molina C, Oram RA. Type 1 diabetes. Lancet. 2018;**391**(10138):2449-2462

[29] Green A, Hede SM, Patterson CC, Wild SH, Imperatore G, Roglic G, et al. Type 1 diabetes in 2017: Global estimates of incident and prevalent cases in children and adults. Diabetologia. 2021;**64**(12):2741-2750

[30] Ogle GD, James S, Dabelea D, Pihoker C, Svennson J, Maniam J, et al. Global estimates of incidence of type 1 diabetes in children and adolescents: Results from the international diabetes federation atlas, 10th edition. Diabetes Research and Clinical Practice. 2022;**183**:109083

[31] Diagnosis and classification of diabetes mellitus. Diabetes Care. 2009;**32**(Suppl. 1):S62-S67. DOI: 10.2337/dc09-s062

[32] Kandemir N, Vuralli D, Ozon A, Gonc N, Ardicli D, Jalilova L, et al. Epidemiology of type 1 diabetes mellitus in children and adolescents: A 50-year,

single-center experience. Journal of Diabetes. 2024;**16**(5):e13562

[33] Streisand R, Monaghan M. Young children with type 1 diabetes: Challenges, research, and future directions. Current Diabetes Reports. 2014;**14**(9):520

[34] International Diabetes Federation. IDF Diabetes Atlas. 10th ed. Brussels, Belgium: International Diabetes Federation; 2021

[35] Sun H, Saeedi P, Karuranga S, Pinkepank M, Ogurtsova K, Duncan BB, et al. IDF diabetes atlas: Global, regional and country-level diabetes prevalence estimates for 2021 and projections for 2045. Diabetes Research and Clinical Practice. 2022;**183**:109119

[36] Ziegler R, Neu A. Diabetes in childhood and adolescence. Deutsches Ärzteblatt International. 2018;**115**(9):146-156

[37] Al-Maskari F, El-Sadig M, Nagelkerke N. Assessment of the direct medical costs of diabetes mellitus and its complications in the United Arab Emirates. BMC Public Health. 2010;**10**:679

[38] Mayer-Davis E, Lawrence J, Dabelea D, Divers J, Isom S, Dolan L, et al. Incidence trends of type 1 and type 2 diabetes among youths, 2002-2012. New England Journal of Medicine. 2017;**376**:1419-1429

[39] Gong B, Yang W, Xing Y, Lai Y, Shan Z. Global, regional, and national burden of type 1 diabetes in adolescents and young adults. Pediatric Research. 2024. DOI: 10.1038/s41390-024-03107-5

[40] Gheith O, Farouk N, Nampoory N, Halim MA, Al-Otaibi T. Diabetic kidney disease: World wide difference of prevalence and risk factors. Journal of Nephropharmacology. 2016;**5**(1):49-56

[41] van Duinkerken E, Snoek FJ, de Wit M. The cognitive and psychological effects of living with type 1 diabetes: A narrative review. Diabetic Medicine. 2020;**37**(4):555-563

[42] Patterson CC, Harjutsalo V, Rosenbauer J, Neu A, Cinek O, Skrivarhaug T, et al. Trends and cyclical variation in the incidence of childhood type 1 diabetes in 26 European centres in the 25 year period 1989-2013: A multicentre prospective registration study. Diabetologia. 2019;**62**(3):408-417

[43] Steck AK, Rewers MJ. Genetics of type 1 diabetes. Clinical Chemistry. 2011;**57**(2):176-185

[44] Al-Balushi M, Al-Badi S, Al-Yaarubi S, Al-Riyami H, Al-Shidhani A, Al-Hinai S, et al. The association of human leukocyte antigens complex with type 1 diabetes in the Omani population. Sultan Qaboos University Medical Journal. 2023;**23**(1):68-75

[45] Knip M, Simell O. Environmental triggers of type 1 diabetes. Cold Spring Harbor Perspectives in Medicine. 2012;**2**(7):a007690

[46] Dashti M, Nizam R, Jacob S, Al-Kandari H, Al Ozairi E, Thanaraj TA, et al. Association between alleles, haplotypes, and amino acid variations in HLA class II genes and type 1 diabetes in Kuwaiti children. Frontiers in Immunology. 2023;**14**. DOI: 10.3389/fimmu.2023.1238269

[47] Noble JA, Valdes AM. Genetics of the HLA region in the prediction of type 1 diabetes. Current Diabetes Reports. 2011;**11**(6):533-542

[48] Bakay M, Pandey R, Hakonarson H. Genes involved in type 1 diabetes: An update. Genes (Basel). 2013;**4**(3):499-521

[49] Redondo MJ, Steck AK, Pugliese A. Genetics of type 1 diabetes. Pediatric Diabetes. 2018;**19**(3):346-353

[50] Ebrahim E, Teklu T, Tajebe F, Wondmagegn T, Akelew Y, Fiseha M. Association of cytotoxic T-lymphocyte antigen-4 gene polymorphism with type 1 diabetes mellitus: In silico analysis of biological features of CTLA-4 protein on Ethiopian population. Diabetes, Metabolic Syndrome and Obesity: Targets and Therapy. 2022;**15**:2733-2751

[51] Huraib GB, Al Harthi F, Arfin M, Al-Asmari A. The protein tyrosine phosphatase non-receptor type 22 (PTPN22) gene polymorphism and susceptibility to autoimmune diseases. In: The Recent Topics in Genetic Polymorphisms. London, UK: IntechOpen; 2020. DOI: 10.5772/intechopen.90836

[52] Armitage LH, Wallet MA, Mathews CE. Influence of PTPN22 Allotypes on innate and adaptive immune function in health and disease. Frontiers in Immunology. 2021;**12**:636618

[53] Rewers M, Ludvigsson J. Environmental risk factors for type 1 diabetes. Lancet. 2016;**387**(10035):2340-2348

[54] Lloyd RE, Tamhankar M, Lernmark Å. Enteroviruses and type 1 diabetes: Multiple mechanisms and factors? Annual Review of Medicine. 2022;**73**:483-499

[55] Coppieters KT, Wiberg A, von Herrath MG. Viral infections and molecular mimicry in type 1 diabetes. APMIS. 2012;**120**(12):941-949

[56] Okada H, Kuhn C, Feillet H, Bach JF. The 'hygiene hypothesis' for autoimmune and allergic diseases: An update. Clinical and Experimental Immunology. 2010;**160**(1):1-9

[57] Cooke A. The hygiene hypothesis and type 1 diabetes. In: Rook GAW, editor. The Hygiene Hypothesis and Darwinian Medicine. Basel: Birkhäuser Basel; 2009. pp. 179-188

[58] Abela AG, Fava S. Association of incidence of type 1 diabetes with mortality from infectious disease and with antibiotic susceptibility at a country level. Acta Diabetologica. 2013;**50**(6):859-865

[59] Infections and vaccinations as risk factors for childhood type I (insulin-dependent) diabetes mellitus: A multicentre case-control investigation. EURODIAB substudy 2 study group. Diabetologia. 2000;**43**(1):47-53. DOI: 10.1007/s001250050006

[60] Xu ZR, Yuan XX, Chen RM, Wei HY, Chen LQ, Du HW, et al. Association between new onset type 1 diabetes and real-world antibiotics and neonicotinoids' exposure-related gut microbiota perturbation. World Journal of Pediatrics. 2022;**18**(10):671-679

[61] Boursi B, Mamtani R, Haynes K, Yang YX. The effect of past antibiotic exposure on diabetes risk. European Journal of Endocrinology. 2015;**172**(6):639-648

[62] Knip M, Virtanen SM, Åkerblom HK. Infant feeding and the risk of type 1 diabetes1234. The American Journal of Clinical Nutrition. 2010;**91**(5):1506S-1513S

[63] Norris JM. Infant and childhood diet and type 1 diabetes risk: Recent advances and prospects. Current Diabetes Reports. 2010;**10**(5):345-349

[64] Lund-Blix NA, Dydensborg Sander S, Størdal K, Nybo Andersen AM,

Rønningen KS, Joner G, et al. Infant feeding and risk of type 1 diabetes in two large Scandinavian birth cohorts. Diabetes Care. 2017;**40**(7):920-927

[65] Miller KM, Hart PH, de Klerk NH, Davis EA, Lucas RM. Are low sun exposure and/or vitamin D risk factors for type 1 diabetes? Photochemical & Photobiological Sciences. 2017;**16**(3):381-398

[66] Samuelsson U, Westerberg L, Aakesson K, Birkebæk N, Bjarnason R, Drivvoll A, et al. Geographical variation in the incidence of type 1 diabetes in the Nordic countries: A study within NordicDiabKids. Pediatric Diabetes. 2019;**21**. DOI: 10.1111/pedi.12943

[67] Taha-Khalde A, Haim A, Karakis I, Shashar S, Biederko R, Shtein A, et al. Air pollution and meteorological conditions during gestation and type 1 diabetes in offspring. Environment International. 2021;**154**:106546

[68] Lodovici M, Bigagli E. Oxidative stress and air pollution exposure. Journal of Toxicology. 2011;**2011**:487074

[69] Jantzen K, Jensen A, Kermanizadeh A, Elholm G, Sigsgaard T, Møller P, et al. Inhalation of house dust and ozone alters systemic levels of endothelial progenitor cells, oxidative stress, and inflammation in elderly subjects. Toxicological Sciences. 2018;**163**(2):353-363

[70] Kurai J, Onuma K, Sano H, Okada F, Watanabe M. Ozone augments interleukin-8 production induced by ambient particulate matter. Genes and Environment. 2018;**40**:14

[71] Holland N, Davé V, Venkat S, Wong H, Donde A, Balmes JR, et al. Ozone inhalation leads to a dose-dependent increase of cytogenetic damage in human lymphocytes. Environmental and Molecular Mutagenesis. 2015;**56**(4):378-387

[72] Vella RE, Pillon NJ, Zarrouki B, Croze ML, Koppe L, Guichardant M, et al. Ozone exposure triggers insulin resistance through muscle c-Jun N-terminal kinase activation. Diabetes. 2015;**64**(3):1011-1024

[73] Tsai DH, Riediker M, Berchet A, Paccaud F, Waeber G, Vollenweider P, et al. Effects of short- and long-term exposures to particulate matter on inflammatory marker levels in the general population. Environmental Science and Pollution Research International. 2019;**26**(19):19697-19704

[74] Bengalli R, Molteni E, Longhin E, Refsnes M, Camatini M, Gualtieri M. Release of IL-1 β triggered by Milan summer PM10: Molecular pathways involved in the cytokine release. BioMed Research International. 2013;**2013**:158093

[75] Bodin J, Stene LC, Nygaard UC. Can exposure to environmental chemicals increase the risk of diabetes type 1 development? BioMed Research International. 2015;**2015**:208947

[76] Gruzieva O, Merid SK, Gref A, Gajulapuri A, Lemonnier N, Ballereau S, et al. Exposure to traffic-related air pollution and serum inflammatory cytokines in children. Environmental Health Perspectives. 2017;**125**(6):067007

[77] Perret JL, Bowatte G, Lodge CJ, Knibbs LD, Gurrin LC, Kandane-Rathnayake R, et al. The dose-response association between nitrogen dioxide exposure and serum Interleukin-6 concentrations. International Journal of Molecular Sciences. 2017;**18**(5). DOI: 10.3390/ijms18051015

[78] Xu J, Huang G, Nagy T, Guo TL. Bisphenol a alteration of type 1 diabetes in non-obese diabetic (NOD) female mice is dependent on window of exposure. Archives of Toxicology. 2019;**93**(4):1083-1093

[79] Ludvigsson J, Andersson-White P, Guerrero-Bosagna C. Toxic metals in cord blood and later development of type 1 diabetes. Pediatric Dimensions. 2019;**4**(2).DOI: 10.15761/pd.1000186

[80] Mauvais-Jarvis F. Gender differences in glucose homeostasis and diabetes. Physiology & Behavior. 2018;**187**:20-23

[81] Blohmé G, Nyström L, Arnqvist HJ, Lithner F, Littorin B, Olsson PO, et al. Male predominance of type 1 (insulin-dependent) diabetes mellitus in young adults: Results from a 5-year prospective nationwide study of the 15-34-year age group in Sweden. Diabetologia. 1992;**35**(1):56-62

[82] Tatti P, Pavandeep S. Gender difference in type 1 diabetes: An underevaluated dimension of the disease. Diabetology. 2022;**3**(2):364-368

[83] Leete P, Mallone R, Richardson SJ, Sosenko JM, Redondo MJ, Evans-Molina C. The effect of age on the progression and severity of type 1 diabetes: Potential effects on disease mechanisms. Current Diabetes Reports. 2018;**18**(11):115

[84] Turtinen M, Härkönen T, Ilonen J, Parkkola A, Knip M. Seasonality in the manifestation of type 1 diabetes varies according to age at diagnosis in Finnish children. Acta Paediatrica. 2022;**111**(5):1061-1069

[85] Nishioka Y, Noda T, Okada S, Myojin T, Kubo S, Higashino T, et al. Incidence and seasonality of type 1 diabetes: A population-based 3-year cohort study using the National Database in Japan. BMJ Open Diabetes Research & Care. 2020;**8**(1):e001262

[86] Spanakis EK, Golden SH. Race/ethnic difference in diabetes and diabetic complications. Current Diabetes Reports. 2013;**13**(6):814-823

[87] Agarwal S, Kanapka LG, Raymond JK, Walker A, Gerard-Gonzalez A, Kruger D, et al. Racial-ethnic inequity in young adults with type 1 diabetes. The Journal of Clinical Endocrinology and Metabolism. 2020;**105**(8):e2960-e2969

[88] Patterson C, Karuranga S, Salpea P, Saeedi P, Dahlquist G, Soltesz G, et al. IDF diabetes atlas: Worldwide estimates of incidence, prevalence and mortality of type 1 diabetes in children and adolescents: Results from the international diabetes federation diabetes atlas, 9th edition. Diabetes Research and Clinical Practice. 2019;**157**:107842

[89] Forga L. The epidemiology of type 1 diabetes: Helping to fit the puzzle pieces. Endocrinología y Nutrición (English Edition). 2015;**62**(4):149-151

[90] Samuelsson U, Westerberg L, Aakesson K, Birkebaek NH, Bjarnason R, Drivvoll AK, et al. Geographical variation in the incidence of type 1 diabetes in the Nordic countries: A study within NordicDiabKids. Pediatric Diabetes. 2020;**21**(2):259-265

[91] Atkinson MA, Eisenbarth GS, Michels AW. Type 1 diabetes. Lancet. 2014;**383**(9911):69-82

[92] Roche EF, McKenna AM, O'Regan M, Ryder KJ, Fitzgerald HM, Hoey HMCV. The incidence of type 1 diabetes in children under 15 years of age is rising again—A nationwide

study. European Journal of Pediatrics. 2023;**182**(10):4615-4623

[93] Dahlquist GG, Nyström L, Patterson CC. Incidence of type 1 diabetes in Sweden among individuals aged 0-34 years, 1983-2007: An analysis of time trends. Diabetes Care. 2011;**34**(8):1754-1759

[94] Lawrence J, Divers J, Isom S, Saydah S, Imperatore G, Pihoker C, et al. Trends in prevalence of type 1 and type 2 diabetes in children and adolescents in the US, 2001-2017. Journal of the American Medical Association. 2021;**326**:717

[95] Ng SM, Soni A. Ten-year review of trends in children with type 1 diabetes in England and Wales. World Journal of Diabetes. 2023;**14**(8):1194-1201

[96] Buchmann M, Tuncer O, Auzanneau M, Eckert AJ, Rosenbauer J, Reitzle L, et al. Incidence, prevalence and care of type 1 diabetes in children and adolescents in Germany: Time trends and regional socioeconomic situation. Journal of Health Monitoring. 2023;**8**(2):57-78

[97] Fox DA, Islam N, Sutherland J, Reimer K, Amed S. Type 1 diabetes incidence and prevalence trends in a cohort of Canadian children and youth. Pediatric Diabetes. 2018;**19**(3):501-505

[98] Miller RG, Secrest AM, Sharma RK, Songer TJ, Orchard TJ. Improvements in the life expectancy of type 1 diabetes: The Pittsburgh epidemiology of diabetes complications study cohort. Diabetes. 2012;**61**(11):2987-2992

[99] Nakhla M, Cuthbertson D, Becker DJ, Pacaud D, Ludvigsson J, Knip M, et al. Diabetic ketoacidosis at the time of diagnosis of type 1 diabetes in children: Insights from TRIGR. JAMA Pediatrics. 2021;**175**(5):518-520

Chapter 3

Type 1 Diabetes: Historical Evolution, Etiological Insights, Pathophysiological Mechanisms, Clinical Manifestations, and Innovative Therapeutic Approaches

Issa Rasheed Fetian, Stefan Zechmann and Lukas Villiger

Abstract

Type 1 diabetes mellitus (T1DM) is a chronic autoimmune condition that results in the destruction of insulin-producing beta cells in the pancreas, finally leading to absolute insulin deficiency. This form of diabetes typically manifests during childhood or adolescence, although it can occur at any age. Unlike type 2 diabetes, which is often associated with lifestyle factors and insulin resistance, type 1 diabetes requires lifelong management through insulin replacement. It has to be said, however, that we are seeing more and more type 1 diabetes in daily practice who, due to their lifestyle and above all obesity, also have insulin resistance in addition to insulin deficiency. This chapter provides a comprehensive overview of type 1 diabetes, including its history, etiology, clinical presentation, diagnosis, and treatment options.

Keywords: type 1 diabetes, historical perspective of diabetes, insulin therapy, blood glucose monitoring, hypoglycemia

1. Introduction

Type 1 diabetes mellitus (T1DM) is an autoimmune disease that leads to the destruction of pancreatic beta cells, finally resulting in an absolute deficiency of insulin [1]. This condition manifests primarily in children and young adults but can occur at any age [2]. The historical understanding of diabetes spans from ancient civilizations, where early symptoms and treatments were described, through the Islamic Golden Age, where significant medical contributions were made by Muslim scholars. Al-Razi (Rhazes) and Avicenna (Ibn Sina) provided early descriptions and insights into diabetes, laying the groundwork for future advancements [3]. The nineteenth century saw the discovery of the role of the pancreas in diabetes, culminating in the breakthrough discovery of insulin in 1921 by Frederick Banting and Charles Best [4].

This chapter reviews the evolution of diabetes management from historical observations to modern treatments, including insulin therapy, glucose monitoring, and emerging therapies such as immunotherapy and gene therapy. By integrating historical perspectives with contemporary research, this chapter aims to provide a thorough understanding of type 1 diabetes and highlight ongoing efforts to improve patient outcomes and quality of life.

2. Historical perspective of diabetes

2.1 Ancient references to diabetes

The earliest known references to diabetes date back to ancient Egypt around 1500 BCE, where the Ebers Papyrus describes a condition characterized by frequent urination. Similar descriptions appear in ancient Indian texts, such as the Charaka Samhita, where a condition called "Madhumeha" (honey urine) is detailed. The sweet smell and taste of urine were notable characteristics that led to the identification of this condition, which we now know as diabetes [5].

In ancient Greece, the physician Aretaeus of Cappadocia (c. first century CE) provided one of the first comprehensive descriptions of diabetes. He described the disease as "a melting down of flesh and limbs into urine," reflecting the severe weight loss and polyuria (excessive urination) associated with the condition. The term "diabetes" is derived from the Greek word "siphon," indicative of the constant passing of urine [6].

2.2 The Islamic Golden Age and contributions by Muslim scientists

The Islamic Golden Age (eighth to fourteenth centuries) marked a significant period of advancement in medicine, including the understanding of diabetes. Muslim scholars played a pivotal role in preserving, translating, and expanding upon the knowledge from ancient civilizations, while also making original contributions (**Figure 1**) [7].

2.2.1 Al-Razi (Rhazes)

Abu Bakr Muhammad ibn Zakariya al-Razi, known in the West as Rhazes (865–925 CE), was a Persian physician who made significant contributions to the medical sciences. In his comprehensive medical encyclopedia, *Kitab al-Hawi fi al-Tibb* (The Comprehensive Book on Medicine), Al-Razi documented his observations of various diseases, including diabetes. He noted the characteristic symptoms of excessive thirst (polydipsia) and urination (polyuria) and was among the first to recognize the presence of sugar in the urine of diabetic patients [8].

2.2.2 Avicenna (Ibn Sina)

Another influential figure in Islamic medicine was Avicenna (980–1037 CE), whose real name was Abu Ali al-Husayn ibn Abdullah ibn Sina. Avicenna's most famous work, *Al-Qanun fi al-Tibb* (The Canon of Medicine), became a cornerstone of medical knowledge in both the Islamic world and Europe. In this text, Avicenna

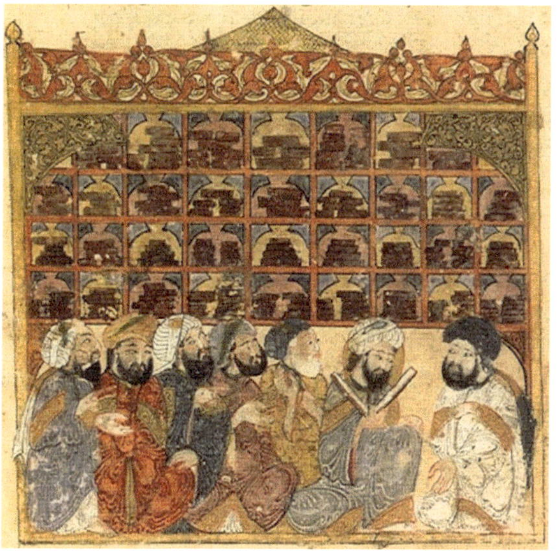

Figure 1.
Painting from Maqamat Hariri, tales written in the twelfth century.

provided detailed descriptions of diabetes, distinguishing between two types of the disease. His account of diabetes mellitus included symptoms such as persistent thirst, excessive urination, and weight loss. He also recognized the potential complications of the disease, such as gangrene, and emphasized the importance of diet in managing the condition [9].

2.2.3 Ibn al-Nafis

Ala-al-Din Abu al-Hassan Ali ibn Abi-Hazm al-Qarshi al-Dimashqi, known as Ibn al-Nafis (1213–1288 CE), made groundbreaking contributions to the understanding of the circulatory system. Although not directly related to diabetes, his work on pulmonary circulation laid important groundwork for future discoveries related to glucose metabolism and the systemic effects of diabetes [10].

2.3 Middle Ages and Renaissance

During the Middle Ages, the understanding of diabetes remained rudimentary, with the disease often diagnosed based on the sweet taste of urine. This method, known as "water tasters," was a crude but effective means of identifying diabetes. The Renaissance period, however, saw a resurgence of interest in scientific inquiry, leading to more systematic observations and the gradual accumulation of medical knowledge.

In the seventeenth century, the English physician Thomas Willis described the sweetness of diabetic urine, coining the term "diabetes mellitus" to distinguish it from other forms of diabetes, such as diabetes insipidus. As previously noticed the word "diabetes" comes from the Greek and means "flowing through," while "mellitus" is derived from the Latin word for honeysweet, reflecting the characteristic sweetness of the urine in this condition [11].

2.4 The nineteenth century: Advances in understanding

Significant advancements in the understanding of diabetes occurred in the nineteenth century. In 1869, German medical student Paul Langerhans discovered clusters of cells in the pancreas, later named the Islets of Langerhans. Although their function was not immediately understood, these cells were later identified as the site of insulin production.

The relationship between the pancreas and diabetes was further elucidated by Oskar Minkowski and Joseph von Mering in 1889. Their experiments demonstrated that removing the pancreas from dogs resulted in severe diabetes, characterized by hyperglycemia and glycosuria. This discovery was pivotal in establishing the pancreas's role in glucose regulation and setting the stage for future research into the treatment of diabetes [12].

2.5 The discovery of insulin

The discovery of insulin in the early twentieth century revolutionized the treatment of type 1 diabetes. In 1921, Canadian scientists Frederick Banting and Charles Best, under the supervision of John Macleod and with the assistance of James Collip, successfully isolated insulin from the pancreas of dogs. This breakthrough demonstrated insulin's ability to lower blood glucose levels in diabetic animals.

The first human patient to receive insulin treatment was Leonard Thompson, a 14-year-old boy with severe diabetes, in 1922. The administration of insulin dramatically improved his condition, transforming diabetes from a fatal disease into a manageable chronic condition. Banting and Macleod were awarded the Nobel Prize in Physiology or Medicine in 1923 for their discovery, and insulin therapy quickly became the standard treatment for type 1 diabetes (**Figure 2**) [13].

2.6 Evolution of diabetes treatment and management

Following the discovery of insulin, the twentieth century saw rapid advancements in diabetes management. The development of long-acting insulin formulations allowed for more stable blood glucose control, while the introduction of insulin syringes and pens made insulin administration more convenient [14].

The advent of home glucose monitoring devices in the 1980s empowered patients to take a more active role in managing their diabetes. This was further enhanced by the development of hemoglobin A1c testing, which provided a more accurate measure of long-term blood glucose control [15].

The twenty-first century has seen further innovations, including continuous glucose monitoring (CGM) systems and closed-loop insulin delivery systems, also known as artificial pancreas systems. These advancements have greatly improved the quality of life for individuals with type 1 diabetes and have reduced the risk of complications associated with poor glucose control [16].

2.7 Understanding type 1 diabetes

The distinction between type 1 and type 2 diabetes became clearer over time, particularly in the mid-twentieth century. Type 1 diabetes was recognized as an autoimmune condition in which the body's immune system attacks and destroys the insulin-producing beta cells in the pancreas. This understanding paved the way

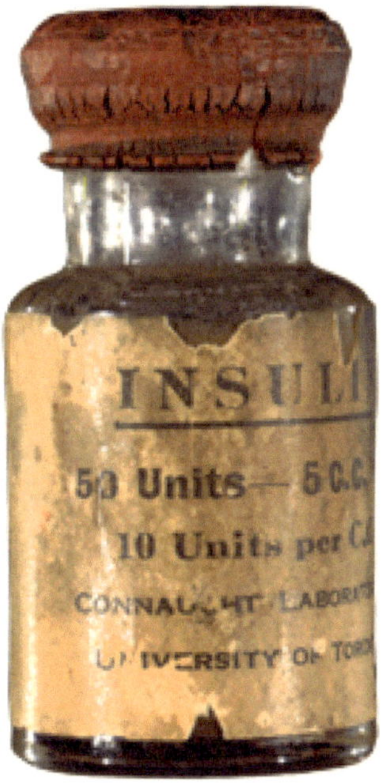

Figure 2.
A bottle of insulin produced at the Connaught Laboratory in Canada.

for research into the immunological aspects of the disease and the development of targeted therapies [17].

Advances in immunology allowed for the identification of autoantibodies associated with type 1 diabetes, further clarifying the disease's autoimmune nature. This understanding has led to ongoing research into potential disease-modifying therapies aimed at halting or preventing the autoimmune attack on beta cells [18].

3. Etiology and pathophysiology of type 1 diabetes

Type 1 diabetes is an autoimmune disease in which the immune system mistakenly targets and destroys the beta cells in the pancreas that produce insulin. The exact cause of this autoimmune response is not fully understood, but it is believed to involve a combination of genetic predisposition and environmental factors [19].

3.1 Genetic factors

Genetics play a significant role in the development of type 1 diabetes. Certain human leukocyte antigen (HLA) genes, particularly those in the HLA-DR and HLA-DQ regions, have been strongly associated with an increased risk of developing the disease. However, not everyone with these genetic markers will develop type 1 diabetes, indicating that other factors must also be involved [20].

3.2 Environmental triggers

Environmental factors are thought to trigger the autoimmune process in genetically predisposed individuals. Possible triggers include viral infections (such as enteroviruses), dietary factors (such as early exposure to cow's milk or gluten), and environmental toxins [21]. The "hygiene hypothesis" suggests that reduced exposure to infectious agents in early childhood might contribute to the development of autoimmune diseases, including type 1 diabetes [22].

3.3 Autoimmune mechanisms

The autoimmune process in type 1 diabetes involves the activation of autoreactive T cells that target and destroy pancreatic beta cells. This process is often marked by the presence of autoantibodies, which can be detected in the blood before the onset of clinical symptoms. The loss of beta cells leads to a progressive decline in insulin production, eventually resulting in the hyperglycemia characteristic of type 1 diabetes (**Figure 3**) [24].

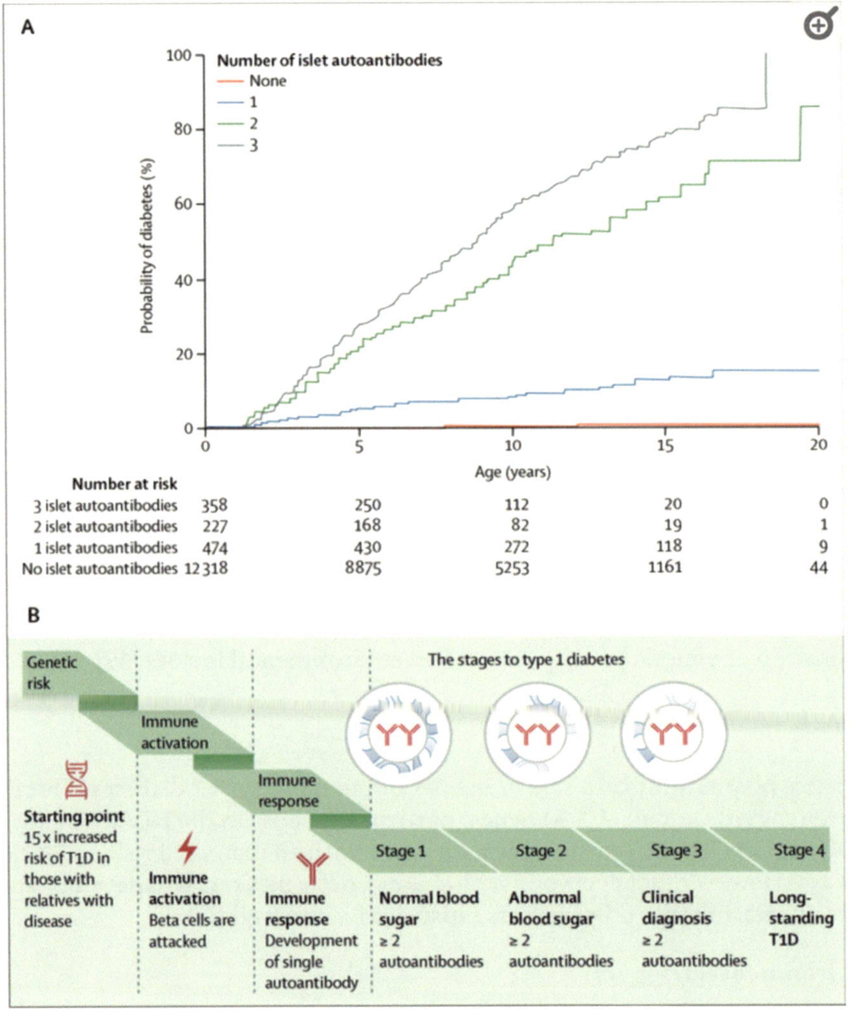

Figure 3.
Factors contributing and disease progression to type 1 diabetes [23].

4. Clinical presentation and diagnosis

4.1 Symptoms

The onset of type 1 diabetes is often sudden, with symptoms appearing over a few weeks. The classic symptoms include the following (**Figure 4**):

- *Polyuria (excessive urination):* Increased glucose in the blood leads to osmotic diuresis, causing frequent urination [25].
- *Polydipsia (excessive thirst):* The loss of fluids due to polyuria leads to dehydration and increased thirst [26].
- *Polyphagia (increased hunger):* Despite high blood glucose levels, the body's cells are starved of energy due to the lack of insulin, leading to increased appetite [27].
- *Weight loss:* The body begins to break down fat and muscle for energy in the absence of insulin, resulting in rapid weight loss [28].
- *Fatigue:* The lack of glucose in cells results in a lack of energy, causing fatigue and weakness [29].
- *Blurred vision:* High blood glucose levels can lead to changes in the lens of the eye, causing blurred vision [30].
- Numbness in the hands or feet: Uncontrolled hyperglycemia paired with several other pathways leads to multiple neurological disorders, with its most classical form the distal symmetric polyneuropathy [31].

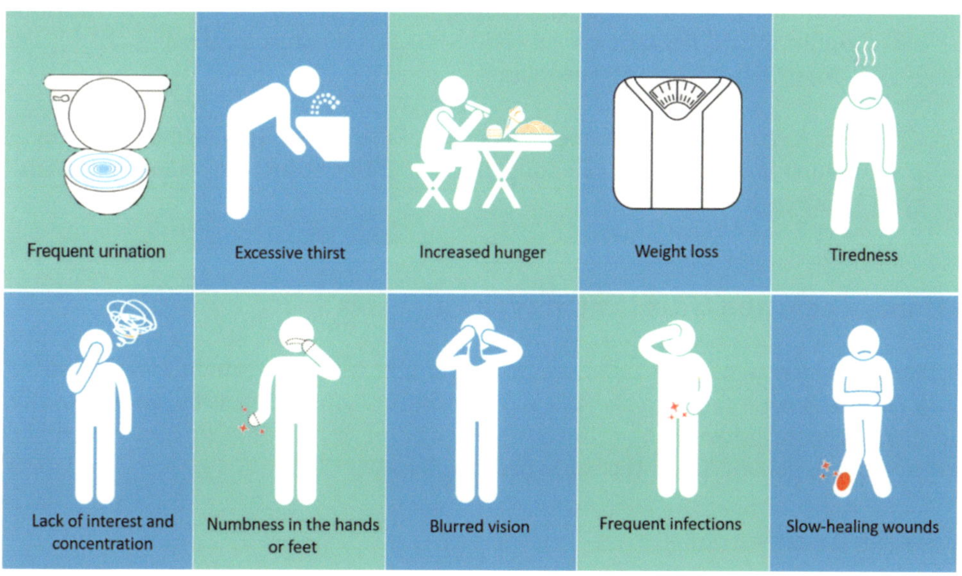

Figure 4.
A visual representation of various diabetic symptoms.

- Slow-healing wounds: Besides other reasons hyperglycemic blood sugar levels induced neuropathy and angiopathy leading to slow-healing wounds and commonly feared diabetic ulcers [32].

- Frequent infections: Uncontrolled hyperglycemic blood sugar levels impair overall immunity leading to an immunocompromised state of diabetic patients *via* involvement of various mechanistic pathways [33].

In some cases, the first sign of type 1 diabetes may be diabetic ketoacidosis (DKA), a life-threatening condition that occurs when the body starts breaking down fats at an excessive rate, leading to the production of ketones and subsequent acidosis [34].

4.2 Diagnosis

The diagnosis of type 1 diabetes is typically confirmed through a combination of clinical presentation and laboratory tests [35]. Key diagnostic criteria include:

- *Fasting plasma glucose (FPG):* A fasting blood glucose level ≥ 126 mg/dL (7.0 mmol/L) is indicative of diabetes.

- *Random plasma glucose:* A random blood glucose level ≥ 200 mg/dL (11.1 mmol/L), along with symptoms of hyperglycemia, is suggestive of diabetes.

- *Hemoglobin A1c (HbA1c):* An HbA1c level ≥ 6.5% indicates chronic hyperglycemia.

- *Autoantibody testing:* The presence of autoantibodies against islet cells, insulin, or glutamic acid decarboxylase (GAD) supports the diagnosis of type 1 diabetes. Four autoantibodies are markers of beta cell autoimmunity in type 1 diabetes: islet cell antibodies (ICA, against cytoplasmic proteins in the beta cell), antibodies to glutamic acid decarboxylase (GAD-65), insulin autoantibodies (IAA), and IA-2A, to protein tyrosine phosphatase.

- *C-peptide levels:* Low or undetectable levels of C-peptide (a marker of insulin production) indicate a lack of endogenous insulin production, consistent with type 1 diabetes.

5. Management and treatment of type 1 diabetes

The primary goal of type 1 diabetes management is to maintain blood glucose levels within a target range to prevent acute complications (such as hypoglycemia and diabetic ketoacidosis) and reduce the risk of long-term complications (such as retinopathy, nephropathy, and cardiovascular disease) [36].

5.1 Insulin therapy

Insulin therapy is the cornerstone of type 1 diabetes management. Various forms of insulin are available, including rapid-acting, short-acting, intermediate-acting, and long-acting insulins. The choice of insulin regimen is tailored to the individual's lifestyle, glucose patterns, and preferences [37]. Insulin can be administered *via*:

- *Syringes or pens*: These are the most common methods of insulin delivery, allowing for multiple daily injections.
- *Insulin pumps:* These devices provide continuous subcutaneous insulin infusion (CSII), allowing for more precise and flexible insulin dosing.
- *Artificial pancreas systems:* These closed-loop systems combine continuous glucose monitoring (CGM) with insulin pumps to automatically adjust insulin delivery based on real-time glucose readings (**Figure 5**).

5.2 Blood glucose monitoring

Regular monitoring of blood glucose levels is essential for effective diabetes management [38]. This can be done through:

- *Self-monitoring of blood glucose (SMBG):* Traditional finger-stick tests provide snapshots of blood glucose levels at specific times.
- *Continuous glucose monitoring (CGM):* CGM systems provide real-time glucose readings, trends, and alerts, helping to prevent hypo- and hyperglycemia.

5.3 Lifestyle management

In addition to insulin therapy, lifestyle management plays a crucial role in type 1 diabetes care [28, 39, 40]. This includes:

- *Diet:* A balanced diet that considers carbohydrate intake is essential for managing blood glucose levels. Patients often work with a dietitian to develop an individualized meal plan. In the course of time and with increasing knowledge, the

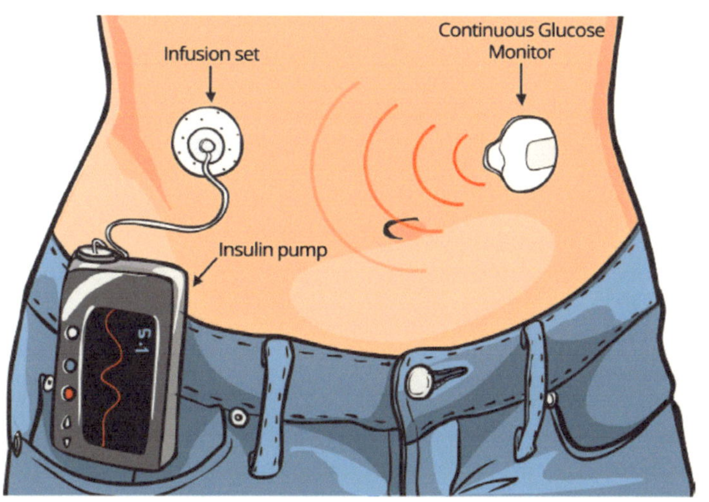

Figure 5.
Modern methods for control blood sugar levels and applying insulin.

patient can then better estimate the carbohydrate content of the food consumed and then apply the necessary insulin dose.

- *Exercise:* Regular physical activity helps improve insulin sensitivity and overall health. However, exercise requires careful monitoring of blood glucose levels to prevent hypoglycemia.

- *Education:* Diabetes education empowers patients to manage their condition effectively, including understanding how to adjust insulin doses, recognize symptoms of hypo- and hyperglycemia, and make informed lifestyle choices. Education and the knowledge that develops from it are the cornerstone for a long and good insulin therapy.

- *Diabetes camp*: Diabetes camps offer an important platform for both education and socialization among pediatric patients with diabetes. These camps, primarily residential, are staffed by healthcare professionals specializing in pediatric diabetes, including nurses, psychologists, and physicians. The camp environment promotes enhanced understanding and acceptance of diabetes among participants, often resulting in improved adherence to glycemic control strategies. To ensure safety, rigorous monitoring of blood glucose levels and precise insulin administration are essential, particularly given the increased physical activity typical of camp settings. This heightened activity necessitates frequent insulin dose adjustments to mitigate the risk of hypoglycemia. The structured and supportive environment of diabetes camps thus plays a crucial role in the effective management of diabetes in children, reinforcing the importance of near-normal glycemic control while addressing the psychosocial aspects of living with diabetes.

5.4 Emerging therapies

Research into type 1 diabetes is ongoing, with several promising areas of investigation, including the following:

- *Immunotherapy:* Approaches aimed at modulating the immune system to halt or slow the autoimmune attack on beta cells are under investigation [41].

- *Islet cell transplantation:* Transplanting healthy islet cells into patients offers the potential for restoring insulin production, though this approach is currently limited by immune rejection and the availability of donor cells [42].

- *Gene therapy:* Experimental gene therapies aim to modify the patient's own cells to produce insulin or protect existing beta cells from autoimmune destruction [43].

5.5 Adjunctive therapies

As mentioned before, insulin was and is the cornerstone of every therapy. Pramlintide is the only non-insulin medication currently approved for improved glycemic control in patients with type 1 diabetes; nonetheless, several other drugs have also been used off-label depending on the patient's need. As mentioned in the abstract, we are seeing more and more type 1 diabetes in daily practice who, due to their lifestyle and above all obesity, also have insulin resistance in addition to insulin deficiency. Due to this fact, they naturally also benefit from therapies that mainly focus on combating insulin resistance. For example, metformin, glucagon-like peptide-1 receptor agonists, dipeptidyl peptidase-4 inhibitors, and sodium-glucose co-transporter-2 (SGLT2) inhibitors have also been used off-label [44].

5.5.1 Complications

Hypoglycemia and ketoacidosis are potentially life-threatening complications, leading to need for assistance from another person in 1 out of 5 patients per leading to hospitalization in 5 out of 100 patients per year, finally causing the deaths of 4–10% of patients with type 1 diabetes [44].

Furthermore, we differentiate between microvascular and macrovascular complications. Microvascular primarily affect eyes (retinopathy), nerves (neuropathy), and the kidney (nephropathy) but can also affect cognitive function, the heart, and other organs [21]. Macrovascular complications cause atherosclerosis and thrombosis in the heart, peripheral arteries, and brain [21].

Books could be filled with the description of the exact pathophysiology, the various forms of these complications and their therapy, so we will leave it here with this very brief and therefore superficial overview.

6. Conclusion

Type 1 diabetes is a complex, lifelong condition that requires careful management to prevent complications and maintain a good quality of life. The history of diabetes, from its earliest descriptions in ancient texts to the groundbreaking discovery of insulin and beyond, reflects the progress that has been made in understanding and treating this disease. Ongoing research continues to seek better treatments and, ultimately, a cure for type 1 diabetes. With advances in technology, education, and therapeutic approaches, individuals with type 1 diabetes can lead full and active lives.

Author details

Issa Rasheed Fetian[1,2,3]*, Stefan Zechmann[4] and Lukas Villiger[5]

1 HAP, Hausarztpraxis, Brugg, Switzerland

2 University of Basel, Basel, Switzerland

3 Acta Klinika, Muttenz, Switzerland

4 Praxis Dr. Zechmann, Winterthur, Switzerland

5 Praxis Dr. Villiger and Diamon Institute, Baden-Dättwil, Switzerland

*Address all correspondence to: issa.fetian@gmail.com

References

[1] Roep BO et al. Type 1 diabetes mellitus as a disease of the β-cell (do not blame the immune system?). Nature Reviews Endocrinology. 2021;**17**(3):150-161

[2] Katsarou A et al. Type 1 diabetes mellitus. Nature Reviews Disease Primers. 2017;**3**(1):1-17

[3] Fleifel M, Fleifel B, El Alam A. Diabetes mellitus across the Arabo-Islamic world: A revolution. International Journal of Endocrinology. 2023;**1**:5541808

[4] Vecchio I et al. The discovery of insulin: An important milestone in the history of medicine. Frontiers in Endocrinology. 2018;**9**:613

[5] Engelhardt D. Diabetes Its Medical and Cultural History. Springer-Verlag Berlin Heidelberg; 1989. ISBN978-3-642-48366-0. DOI: 10.1007/978-3-642-48364-6

[6] Gale E. Life in the Age of Insulin. Cham: Springer; 2024

[7] Hajar R. The air of history part III: The golden age in Arab islamic medicine: An introduction. Heart Views. 2013;**14**(1):43-46

[8] Amr SS, Tbakhi A. Abu Bakr Muhammad Ibn Zakariya Al Razi (Rhazes): Philosopher, physician and alchemist. Annals of Saudi Medicine. 2007;**27**(4):305-307

[9] Gutas D. Ibn Sina [Avicenna]. In: The Stanford Encyclopedia of Philosophy. 15 Sep 2016. Available from: https://plato.stanford.edu/archives/win2024/entries/ibn-sina/

[10] West JB. Ibn al-Nafis, the pulmonary circulation, and the Islamic golden age. Journal of Applied Physiology. 2008;**105**(6):1877-1880

[11] Thompson RP. Theories and Models in Medicine, Philosophy of Medicine. London: Taylor and Francis Group; 2011. pp. 115-136

[12] Lambert C, Delgado E. 100 years since the discovery of insulin, from its discovery to the insulins of the future. Biomedicine. 2024;**12**(3):533

[13] Bliss M. The Discovery of Insulin. Historica Canada: The Canadian Encyclopedia; 2015. Article; Last Edited November 08, 2023

[14] Bolli GB, Cheng AYY, Owens DR. Insulin: Evolution of insulin formulations and their application in clinical practice over 100 years. Acta Diabetologica. 2022;**59**(9):1129-1144

[15] Weinstock RS, Aleppo G, Bailey TS, et al. The Role of Blood Glucose Monitoring in Diabetes Management. Arlington (VA): American Diabetes Association; 2020. DOI: 10.2337/db2020-31. Available from: https://www.ncbi.nlm.nih.gov/books/NBK566165/

[16] Kropff J, Hans DeVries J. Continuous glucose monitoring, future products, and update on worldwide artificial pancreas projects. Diabetes Technology and Therapeutics. 2016;**18**(S2):S2-S53

[17] Krause M, De Vito G. Type 1 and type 2 diabetes mellitus: Commonalities, differences and the importance of exercise and nutrition. Nutrients. 2023;**15**(19):4279

[18] Noble JA, Erlich HA. Genetics of type 1 diabetes. Cold Spring

Harbor Perspectives in Medicine. 2012;**2**(1):a007732

[19] Houeiss P, Luce S, Boitard C. Environmental triggering of type 1 diabetes autoimmunity. Frontiers in Endocrinology. 2022;**13**:933965

[20] Lee HS, Hwang JS. Genetic aspects of type 1 diabetes. Annals of Pediatric Endocrinology and Metabolism. 2019;**24**(3):143

[21] Lyons SK, Hermann JM, Miller KM, et al. Use of adjuvant pharmacotherapy in type 1 diabetes: International comparison of 49,996 individuals in the prospective diabetes follow-up and T1D exchange registries. Diabetes Care. 2017;**40**:e139-e140

[22] Rewers M, Ludvigsson J. Environmental risk factors for type 1 diabetes. The Lancet. 2016;**387**(10035):2340-2348

[23] Syed FZ. Type 1 "diabetes mellitus". Annals of Internal Medicine. 2022;**175**(3):ITC33-ITC48. DOI: 10.7326/AITC202203150. Epub 2022 Mar 8

[24] Burrack AL, Martinov T, Fife BT. T cell-mediated beta cell destruction: Autoimmunity and alloimmunity in the context of type 1 diabetes. Frontiers in Endocrinology. 2017;**8**:343

[25] Spira A, Gowrishankar M, Halperin ML. Factors contributing to the degree of polyuria in a patient with poorly controlled diabetes mellitus. American Journal of Kidney Diseases. 1997;**30**(6):829-835

[26] Kotagiri R, Kutti Sridharan G. Primary polydipsia [Updated: July 24, 2023]. In: StatPearls [Internet]. Treasure Island (FL): StatPearls Publishing; Jan 2025. Available from: https://www.ncbi.nlm.nih.gov/books/NBK562251/

[27] Röder PV et al. Pancreatic regulation of glucose homeostasis. Experimental and Molecular Medicine. 2016;**48**(3):e219-e219

[28] Gan MJ, Albanese-O'Neill A, Haller MJ. Type 1 diabetes: Current concepts in epidemiology, pathophysiology, clinical care, and research. Current Problems in Pediatric and Adolescent Health Care. 2012;**42**(10):269-291

[29] Kalra S, Sahay R. Diabetes fatigue syndrome. Diabetes Therapy. 2018;**9**:1421-1429

[30] Ghimire P, Dhamoon AS, Doerr C. Ketoacidosis (Nursing) [Updated: August 8, 2023]. In: StatPearls [Internet]. Treasure Island (FL): StatPearls Publishing; Jan 2025. Available from: https://www.ncbi.nlm.nih.gov/books/NBK568717/, https://www.cdc.gov/diabetes/diabetes-complications/diabetes-and-vision-loss.html

[31] Davis WA, Hamilton E, Davis TME. Temporal trends in distal symmetric polyneuropathy in type 2 diabetes: The fremantle diabetes study. The Journal of Clinical Endocrinology and Metabolism. 2024;**109**(3):e1083-e1094. DOI: 10.1210/clinem/dgad646

[32] Margolis DJ, Kantor J, Santanna J, Strom BL, Berlin JA. Risk factors for delayed healing of neuropathic diabetic foot ulcers: A pooled analysis. Archives of Dermatology. 2000;**136**(12):1531-1535. DOI: 10.1001/archderm.136.12.1531

[33] Holt RIG, Cockram CS, Ma RCW, Luk AOY. Diabetes and infection: Review of the epidemiology, mechanisms and principles of treatment. Diabetologia. 2024;**67**(7):1168-1180. DOI: 10.1007/s00125-024-06102-x. Epub 2024 Feb 20

[34] American Diabetes Association. Diagnosis and classification of

diabetes mellitus. Diabetes Care. 2010;**33**(1):S62-S69

[35] Subramanian S, Baidal D. The management of type 1 diabetes [Updated: May 22, 2021]. In: Feingold KR, Ahmed SF, Anawalt B, et al., editors. Endotext [Internet]. South Dartmouth (MA): MDText.com, Inc.; 2000. Available from: https://www.ncbi.nlm.nih.gov/books/NBK279114/

[36] Thota S, Akbar A. Insulin [Updated: July 10, 2023]. In: StatPearls [Internet]. Treasure Island (FL): StatPearls Publishing; Jan 2024. Available from: https://www.ncbi.nlm.nih.gov/books/NBK560688/

[37] Fetian IR, Maziukas R, Pisarcikova Z, Zechmann S, Dolinar M, Dolinar S, et al. “Bathtub” shape is a key term for interpreting the course of blood glucose curves. Healthbook TIMES Das Schweizer Ärztejournal Journal Des Médecins Suisses. 2025;**5**(1-2):98-104

[38] Ahmad F, Joshi SH. Self-care practices and their role in the control of diabetes: A narrative review. Cureus. 2023;**15**(7):e41409. DOI: 10.7759/cureus.41409

[39] Fetian IR. Unveiling the Significance of the ‘Bathtub’ Shape in Blood Glucose Curve Analysis. London, UK: IntechOpen; 2024. DOI: 10.5772/intechopen.1003746

[40] Nigam S et al. Nanotechnology in immunotherapy for type 1 diabetes: Promising innovations and future advances. Pharmaceutics. 2022;**14**(3):644

[41] Bruni A et al. Islet cell transplantation for the treatment of type 1 diabetes: Recent advances and future challenges. Diabetes, Metabolic Syndrome and Obesity: Targets and therapy. 2014;**7**:211-223

[42] El Nahas R, Al-Aghbar MA, Herrero L, van Panhuys N, Espino-Guarch M. Applications of genome-editing Technologies for Type 1 diabetes. International Journal of Molecular Sciences. 2023;**25**(1):344. DOI: 10.3390/ijms25010344

[43] Åkerblom HK, Knip M. Putative environmental factors in type 1 diabetes. Diabetes/Metabolism Reviews. 1998;**14**(1):31-68

[44] DiMeglio LA, Evans-Molina C, Oram RA. Type 1 diabetes. Lancet. 2018;**16**(391):2449-2462. DOI: 10.1016/S0140-6736(18)31320-5

Section 2

Current Treatment and Management

Chapter 4

Current Pharmacological Treatments in Type 1 Diabetes and Patient Tolerability against New Generation Medicines

Muzaffer Serdar Deniz

Abstract

Type 1 diabetes mellitus (T1D) is an autoimmune condition characterized by insulin deficiency due to pancreatic beta-cell destruction. The global incidence of T1D has been increasing and reached 12 million patients in 2021. Diabetes is expected to rank third place, following cardiovascular disease and stroke within factors that reduce life expectancy. T1D patients suffer from poor glycemic control due to fluctuations in glucose levels, leading to cardiovascular disease, nephropathy, and retinopathy. T1D currently has no cure, and management strategies are crucial for improving the quality of patient life. In this chapter, we will be discussing advancements in diabetes technologies, focusing on management and emerging therapies. Newer technologies in glucose monitoring, better analogs for insulin replacement therapies, and advanced continuous subcutaneous insulin infusion (CSII) devices eliminating the burden of manual multiple daily injections (MDI) are proving to be beneficial to diabetics. Additionally, combined adjunct therapies where amylin analogs, GLP-1 receptor agonists, and SGLT2 inhibitors, as well as emerging immunotherapy, offer complementary benefits in managing T1D. Although surgical interventions such as the pancreas or islet transplantations are currently applied as a necessary measure to rescue organ failure, advancements in stem cell technologies and synthetic biology eliminate donor requirements and increase the survival of transplants.

Keywords: type 1 diabetes, glucose monitoring, insulin replacement, diabetes technologies, adjunct therapy, transplantation

1. Introduction

Diabetes mellitus (DM) is a chronic disorder where insulin production from pancreas beta cells is limited or lacking [1]. Insulin hormone is vital for glucose uptake from the circulation to the cells for energy metabolism. Type 1 diabetes (T1D) is a form of DM where the insulin-producing beta cells are destroyed and the insulin production is diminished [1]. In a global disease burden projection study, DM is recognized as a health burden globally and determined as the third major leading factor that reduces life expectancy in 2022–2050 [2]. In 2021, the statistics revealed approximately 8.4 million T1D patients, reaching 12 million with missing prevalence, especially in the sub-Saharan region. Of those, 18% were children younger than 20 years old, and 64% were diagnosed later in life, age 20–59 [3]. The incidence is 40 per 100,000 people annually, increasing by 3–4% yearly, varying throughout regions [3, 4]. In Europe, specifically in Poland and Finland, pediatric T1D incidence increased by 11–15% between 1994 and 2022 [5]. This trend in DM incidence urges us to develop and adapt better approaches for diagnosis, care, and management of DM.

The mechanisms involved in the T1D pathogenesis are the generation of autoantibodies [4] and autoreactive T cells [6] against insulin-producing pancreatic beta-cells. T1D has a strong genetic component; however, only 10% of the patients have a family history of T1D [7]. The T1D risk in adolescents without family history is calculated as 1:300, and the risk increases to 1:50 for maternal and 1:15 in case of paternal genetic burden [8]. Although the disease pathology cannot be attributed to a single gene or a variant [9], there are 75 genetic risk loci identified [10], including major histocompatibility complex (MHC), INVR associated with insulin action, and genes related to immune regulation (CTLA4, GATA6, FOXP3, etc.) [1, 7, 9, 10]. On the other hand, environmental factors such as infections, chemicals, and dietary factors are often attributed to environmental components of T1D [8].

The levels of autoantibodies against insulin, glutamic acid decarboxylase (GAD), protein tyrosine phosphatase IA-2 or IA-2, and zinc transporter 8 (ZnT8) in the serum determine the disease onset and are mainly detected in children who are younger than 10 years old [11]. Following the progression of the T1D, stage 2 is marked by dysglycemia or glucose intolerance and remains asymptomatic. The symptomatic disease stage, stage 3, persists with the clinical representation of hyperglycemia and might be coupled with diabetic ketoacidosis (DKA) or diabetic hyperosmolar syndrome [1, 6, 12]. Poor management of blood glucose levels in the absence of insulin may later cause more systemic health problems, including cardiovascular diseases, retinopathy, and nephropathy, and reduce life expectancy [13].

In the clinic, DM is diagnosed by symptoms such as hyperglycemia, polydipsia, polyuria, weight loss, fatigue, and blurred vision coupled with laboratory tests measuring serum glucose, autoantibody, and insulin levels [1, 12]. There is no cure for DM; however, (i) early diagnosis and (ii) consistent management are crucial for preventing complications and maintaining a good quality of life for individuals with T1D [14]. This book chapter will focus on the advancements in diabetes technology, including the devices and treatment approaches for blood glucose monitoring, insulin and non-insulin-based adjuvant therapies, and surgical approaches.

2. Glucose monitoring

The T1D management strategies focus on diet, physical activity, and glucose level monitoring [1, 12, 14]. Particularly, blood glucose monitoring, either real-time or self-monitoring, is essential for glycemic management [15]. Hemoglobin A1c (HbA1c) is a golden standard for determining glycemic status over a 2–3-month period and is more powerful when combined with glycemic variability (GV) collected from individual patients [16]. The main goal in clinics for T1D patients, whether they are children or adults, is to maintain hemoglobin A1c (HbA1c) below 53 mmol/mol

(7%) [17]. More specifically, the time in range (TIR) should be between 70 and 180 mg/dL / 3.9–10 mmol/L while minimizing both time below range (TBR) and time above range (TAR) to 4 and 25%, respectively, to keep the glucose level fluctuations minimal [17]. Glucose monitoring technology enables patients to make informed decisions and real-time adjustments to their diet, physical activity, insulin, and medication intake, preventing undesirable health conditions such as diabetic ketoacidosis and glycemic attacks [15]. Also, the read-out of the glucose levels provides valuable information to determine the habits of the particular patients and provide patient-specific regimens for diabetes management [15, 18].

2.1 Self-monitoring of blood glucose

Self-monitoring of blood glucose (SMBG) involves individuals regularly monitoring their blood glucose levels using a device called a glucometer. This process typically requires a small blood sample, usually obtained through a finger prick [15, 18, 19]. The SMBG device measures the glucose levels by an electrochemical method where the glucose is oxidized by glucose oxidase or glucose dehydrogenase with a coenzyme and reads voltage semi-quantitatively [19]. The patients measure their blood glucose before and after meals daily and identify patterns of improvements to their management and therapy protocols [15]. SBGM is a beneficial tool, especially for T1D patients receiving insulin therapies [15, 20]. The most important limitation of SMBG is the collection of the blood glucose profile of a specific moment, making it challenging to capture particularly the postprandial and nocturnal blood glucose levels [21].

2.2 Continuous glucose monitoring

Continuous glucose monitoring (CGM) systems use a transdermal sensor to measure glucose levels continuously. CGM devices have three components: the sensor, which carries out the glucose measurement; the transmitter, which collects the sensor readings; and the receiver, to read the glucose measurement [22]. Similar to SMBG devices, the CGM sensor also determines the glucose levels by (i) electrochemical, (ii) optical, (iii) thermal, or (iv) physicochemical methods [22]. One of the main differences between SMBG and CGM devices is that CGM measures glucose levels in interstitial fluid, whereas SMBG devices collect data from blood glucose levels [15, 19, 22]. Although the blood and interstitial fluid glucose levels are well correlated, due to glucose uptake to the tissue and cells, the readings from the interstitial fluid are delayed for approximately 5–15 minutes compared to the blood measurements [22]. Nevertheless, overall, CGM devices provide real-time glucose readings and trends throughout the day and night. This improves glycemic control and reduces the discomfort of finger pricks [22, 23].

2.2.1 Continuous glucose monitoring

The CGM device technology is based on two types of devices: (i) real-time (rtCGM) and (ii) flash, intermittent scanned (isCGM) CGM devices [22, 24]. rtCGM consists of three components described above, providing continuous, real-time measurements and hypoglycemia and hyperglycemia alarms. Whereas isCGM devices have a combined sensor and transmitter but require the user to scan the sensor to obtain information manually and lack alarms [24].

	FreeStyle Libre 2	FreeStyle Libre 3	Dexcom G6	Dexcom G7	Medtronic Guardian 3	Medtronic Guardian 4	Eversense E3
Type of system	isCGM	rtCGM	rtCGM	rtCGM	rtCGM	rtCGM	rtCGM
FDA-approved sites	Arm	Arm	Abdomen	Abdomen or arm	Abdomen or arm	Abdomen or arm	Arm (implanted subcutaneously)
Sensor wear	14 days	14 days	10 days	10 days	7 days	7 days	180 days
Warm-up time	1 hour	1 hour	2 hours	30 minutes	2 hours	2 hours	24 hours
Method of insertion	Self-insertion	Self-insertion	Self-insertion	Self-insertion	Self-insertion	Self-insertion	Requires office-based procedure
Calibration required?	No	No	No	No	Yes, every 12 hours (3 to 4 times recommended)	No	Yes, every 12 hours for the first 21 days of use, then once daily
Active automatic alerts	Low and High	Low and High	Predictive low and high, rate of change, low and high	Predictive low and high, rate of change, low and high	Predictive low and high, rate of change, low and high	Predictive low and high, rate of change, low and high	Predictive low and high, rate of change, low and high
Programmed/ Mandatory alarms for glucose values	None	Urgent Low	Urgent Low	Urgent Low	Urgent Low	Urgent Low	Urgent Low
Ability to use Hybrid Closed closed-loop therapy when Integrated pump	None	None	Tandem t: X2 and Omnipod 5	No (in development)	Medtronic MiniMed 670G, 770G, 780G	Medtronic MiniMed 780G	No
Share feature for healthcare providers	LibreView	LibreView	Clarity	Clarity	CareLink	CareLink	Eversense Data Management System (DMS) Pro
Affected by medications	No	Yes, Vitamin C	No	Yes, Hydroxyurea	Yes, Paracetamol	Yes, Paracetamol	Yes, Mannitol, Tetracycline

Table 1.
Personal CGM devices commonly used in the United States. (Sanchez et al. [34]).

Studies clearly showed that CGM device use has a beneficial effect on diabetes management. A recent study focusing on the benefits of CGM devices in managing both T1D and type 2 diabetes (T2D) revealed that real-time CGM use was associated with significantly lower HbA1c and rates of emergency department visits or hospitalizations for hypoglycemia [23]. Regardless, the meta-analysis of the literature further demonstrated that regardless of the type of diabetes, CGM device use, both professional [25] and personal [26], is associated with greater HbA1c reduction from baseline, improving glycemic control by expanding TIR and decreasing TBR, TAR, and glucose variability [25, 26].

Japanese cohorts focusing on the efficacy of isCGM vs. SMBG devices in diabetes management demonstrated clearly that isCGM device measurement correlated well with SMBG [21] and the isCGM use is associated with better HbA1c levels and lower hospitalization due to glycemic attack [27]. Nevertheless, another study compared the efficacy of rtCGM vs. isCGM devices in controlling glycemia in T1D patients, data derived from CORRIDA randomized trials. The study describes that rtCGM was superior in reducing hypoglycemia and improving TIR with normal hypoglycemia awareness during 4 days of intensive physical activity. The beneficial effect was attributed to the alarm system of rtCGM devices [28].

CGM devices are beneficial technology; however, there are underreported issues associated with transdermal sensors of CGM, such as skin irritations [29, 30], infections [29], allergic reactions [31], and cutaneous trauma [29]. Those reports indicate the need for further improvements regarding patient experience by reducing skin-based discomforts.

Overall, CGM devices are beneficial for individuals who have great GV, which presents as hyperglycemia or hypoglycemia, struggle to maintain HbA1c levels, and need detailed and continuous glucose monitoring. Professional CGM is valuable for clinical evaluations and making informed treatment decisions, while personal CGM enables patients to manage their condition more effectively.

2.2.2 Continuous glucose monitoring report evaluation

The CGM data became crucial in diabetes treatment approaches by providing personalized solutions to individual DM cases and enhancing the data pool for further use in disease projections. To collect this valuable information, metric factors such as glucose measurements, timelines, along with environmental conditions should be evaluated [32]. In detail, the glycemic variability, including TIR, TAR, and TBR values, mean glucose levels, lowest and highest blood glucose indexes, and estimated HbA1c levels data were collected; during the time the CGM device was active and worn [32, 33]. The 2017 consensus provides numerical values for the standardized CGM metrics to evaluate the effectiveness of the treatment approach and regimen on a patient basis [32, 33]. Further comprehensive real-world data from the USA on CGM device use provided the efficacy and accuracy of the particular CGM devices according to the standardized CGM parameters (**Table 1**) [34].

3. T1 DM management

3.1 Insulin therapy

DM arises from insulin production deficiency. The main treatment approach is providing an external insulin source to the patients to maintain their glycemic status. The discovery of insulin is a key achievement in medical history and was awarded the Nobel Prize in 1923 to Benting and McLeod [35, 36]. Benting and Best isolated Langerhans' cells, identified previously by a German medical student, Paul Langerhans, in 1869, and transferred the isolate to the diabetic dogs. Following their successful interventions, with the assistance of Collip and Macleod, the team carried out the first and successful transfer of the purified Langerhans' isolate to a 14-year-old diabetic, improving his condition significantly [35, 36]. The discovery of Benting and colleagues further adapted to commercially available products. The first commercial insulin was a protamine zinc insulin with delayed response adsorption and extended action during the 1930s, but it presented great instability. In 1946s, neutral protamine Hagedorn (NPH), premixed with soluble insulin, became the primary basal insulin throughout the twentieth century. In the 1980s, the first human insulin development was followed by the production of insulin analogs such as glargine and detemir, which demonstrated less day-to-day variability and a longer duration of action, allowing for once-daily dosing [36, 37].

The advances in diabetes technology are intertwined with the molecular characterization of insulin [36]. Adapting the newest technologies, preliminary pork then the beef pancreas, became the source of insulin purification. Additionally, better purification techniques enable the collection of more concentrated insulin, from 5 U (units/mL) up to 100 U in the 1980s [36, 38].

The efficacy of exogenous insulin administration largely depends on the pharmacokinetics of the insulin isolate or the analog. The regular insulin poorly mimicked endogenous insulin due to self-forming hexamers upon entry into the bloodstream, which delayed the response by approximately 60–90 minutes. Within the body, insulin is produced as pre-insulin and processed to dimers and monomers to facilitate entry into the cells. Thus, advances in molecular techniques shift the technology from insulin purification from the animal pancreas to recombinant human insulin production with long-lasting effects and faster adsorption [36]. According to the needs of patients, two classes of insulin analogs, Bolus vs. Basal insulin analogs, are currently available. Bolus insulin products are rapid-acting insulin analogs (RAA), including insulin lispro, aspart, and glulisine, used to counteract postprandial glucose (PPG) excursions [39, 40]. On the other hand, basal insulin analogs are long-acting, such as insulin glargine, detemir, and degludec, and are used primarily to manage fasting plasma glucose levels [25, 39].

3.1.1 Bolus insulin products

RAA is taken shortly before mealtime to adjust the PPG and prevent hyperglycemia. Lispro and Aspart, two main Bolus analogs, adsorbed within 10–20 minutes, and their effects last up to 7 hours (**Table 2**) [41]. Due to their rapid dissociation, multiple administration is needed daily (MDI) to maintain the glycemic status. The new generation "Ultra-Rapid Acting Insulin Analog (URAA)" was designed to mimic better the endogenous insulin mode of action [40, 41]. These URAA analogs called faster aspart (URAsp) and insulin lispro-aabc (URLi) produced by the addition of compounds such as niacinamide [42] and L-arginine [40, 43].

The URLi was designed with the addition of treprostinil and citrate [44, 45] to enhance vasodilation and vascular permeability, respectively. The two double-blinded studies assessing the efficacy of URLi to its slower version, Lispro analog, clearly demonstrated faster adsorption and 3–5-fold greater insulin action regardless

PREPARATIONS	ONSET	PEAK	DURATION
1. BOLUS INSULIN PRODUCTS			
1.A. An ultra-rapid acting			
Faster aspart	16–20 min.	63 min.	5–7 hours
Insulin lispro-aabc	15–17 min.	57 min	4,6–7,3 hours
Insulin human-inhaled	12 min.	35–40 min.	90–180 min.
1.B. Rapid-acting analog			
Insulin aspart	10–20 min.	30–90 min.	3–5 hours
Insulin lispro			
Insulin glulisine			
1.C. Short-acting			
Regular	30–60 min.	2–4 hours	5–8 hours
2.BASAL INSULIN PRODUCTS			
2.A. Intermediate-acting			
NPH	2–4 hours	4–10 hours	10–24 hours
2.B. Long-acting analog			
Insulin detemir	1,5–4 hours	6–14 hours	16–20 hours
Insulin glargine (U-100)	2–4 hours	No peak	20–24 hours
Insulin glargine (U-300)	6 hours	No peak	36 hours
Insulin degludec (U-100, U-200)	1 hour	No peak	42 hours
3.COMBINATION PRODUCTS			
70% NPH/30% regular	30–60 min.	Dual	10–16 hours
75% NPL, 25% lispro	5–15 min.	Dual	10–16 hours
50% NPL, 50% lispro	5–15 min.	Dual	10–16 hours
70% insulin aspart protamine	5–15 min.	Dual	15–18 hours

Table 2.
Pharmacodynamics of insulin preparations.

of the type of diabetes [45], and the URLi effect was maintained throughout different doses [44]. Further studies suggested that using URLi mealtimes to adjust postprandial glucose, combined with a basal insulin regimen, is optimal for glycemic control [46–48].

3.1.2 Basal insulin products

Basal insulin analogs are long-acting insulin analogs (LAA) designed to manage fasting glucose levels with long-lasting effects for up to 42 hours [36]. The first designed analog was insulin glargine around the 2000s. Changing the amino acid composition of the detemir analog shifted its isoelectric point so that precipitates at neutral pH contribute to its slow disassociation at the side of injection [49]. Glargine insulin demonstrated comparable glucose level reduction capacity. However, glargine was better at reducing hypoglycemic risk in a randomized trial with NPH [50]. The glargine insulin produced two different concentrations, Gla-100 U (100 units/mL) and Gla-300 U (300 units/mL). Randomized trials focused on the efficacy of the dose for glycemic control in DM patients from Japan [51], and a meta-analysis of the literature [52] found that regardless of the type of DM, Gla-100 and Gla-300 have comparable efficacy and safety; however, Gla-300 presented enhanced nocturnal glycemic control. The Gla-300 efficacy and safety were also replicated in another cohort composed of children and adolescent diabetics [53].

Detemir was the next LAA designed around 2005, and it had a side chain and an increased affinity to albumin, facilitating its long-lasting effect [54]. Ten years later, another analog, insulin degludec, has been produced. Degludec insulin forms a depot of multi-hexamers at the side injection which increases the disassociation interval up to 42 hours [55].

The clinical trials compare the efficacy and safety of different types of LAA, which is crucial for determining the strengths and weaknesses of particular regimens, thus providing valuable information to improve patient care. The two studies comparing the efficacy of Gla-300 and Degludec-100 in T1D patients showed comparable changes in the HbA1c, nocturnal glucose, and hypoglycemia [56], a more drastic changes observed in real-time glucodensity and nocturnal glucose levels [57]. According to the efficacy and safety data, an updated regimen for T1D management is summarized in **Table 3**.

3.2 Insulin delivery systems: continuous subcutaneous insulin infusion (CSII, insulin pump)

The widely used treatment option for T1D is the insulin replacement therapy. Evolving technologies offer an alternate system to induce insulin exogenously. Continuous subcutaneous insulin infusion (CSII) is a method where insulin is delivered to the patient *via* an insulin pump [58, 59]. The development of insulin pumps dates back to the 1970s, and the more modern versions are used in 40–60% of T1D patients in Western countries [60]. Although the clinical studies showed a comparable outcome regarding glycemic control [61, 62], the automated injections of multiple daily insulin doses became more convenient, and their use has expanded among DM patients [63]. The traditional insulin pumps deliver either bolus or basal insulin through a catheter inserted subcutaneously [58]. Types of insulin pumps can be categorized under three main subjects: (i) traditional insulin pumps, (ii) patch pumps, and (iii) hybrid closed-loop systems.

Insulin regimens	Compliance	Reduced hypoglycemia risk	Increased costs
MDI with LAA + RAA or URAA	+++	+++	+++
Secondary Injected Regimens (Less-Preferred)			
MDI with NPH + RAA or URAA	++	++	++
MDI with NPH + short-acting (regular) insulin	++	+	+
Two daily injections with NPH + short-acting (regular) insulin or premixed	+	+	+

Table 3.
Types of insulin regimens for managing T1DM.

Traditional insulin pumps consist of a cannula connected to the insulin reservoir via line tubing. The traditional pump facilitates the MDI of either basal or bolus insulin. The delivery intervals and the dose can be adjusted manually [58, 63]. Patch pumps were introduced around 15 years ago as the tubeless alternative to traditional pumps, where a patch containing an insulin reservoir was inserted subcutaneously, and the release was managed by a handheld device [64].

The closed-loop system of insulin delivery combined with a CGM device [65]. Starting from the earlier versions of more advanced forms of the system are sensor-augmented pumps (SAP), hybrid closed-loop systems, and advanced hybrid closed-loop systems (artificial pancreas), respectively. Sensor-augmented insulin pumps combine CGM with insulin pump therapy, providing real-time glucose data so that patients make informed adjustments to insulin delivery. SAP minimizes the risk of hypoglycemia. Clinical trials comparing MDI vs. SAP use found that SAP effectively lowers HbA1c [66, 67] up to 18 months follow-up phase [66]. Closed-loop systems, also known as hybrid closed-loop systems, automatically adjust basal insulin delivery based on CGM readings, thus improving all-day TIRs and TBRs, reducing the burden of manual adjustments, and improving glucose control [68]. Clinical trials with a smaller sample pool demonstrated that during the hybrid closed-loop delivery system, no severe hypoglycemia or ketoacidosis was recorded [69], and it is safe to use at home [70].

The artificial pancreas is an advanced form of insulin-only, single-hormone delivery system [65]. The artificial pancreas continuously monitors glucose levels and automatically administers both basal and bolus insulin doses as needed, closely mimicking the insulin regulation by the pancreas [71]. The process holds in real time and thus can predict and prevent hypoglycemia by suspending or reducing insulin, during sleep or physical activity [59, 65].

Two hormones, insulin and glucagon, regulate glucose metabolism. Insulin induces glucose uptake into the cells, lowering blood glucose, while glucagon directs the release of stored glucose, raising blood glucose levels [72]. Due to the dual mechanism of the pancreas, single-hormone-based treatment approaches fall short of managing hypoglycemia properly [73]. A state-of-the-art invention, bionic pancreas trials are ongoing [74]. This system adjusts and administers insulin and glucagon when needed, closely replicating the pancreas's function. Specifically, glucagon delivery reacts to glucose level reduction and counters hypoglycemia [59, 74].

3.3 Non-insulin treatment and adjunct therapies

Insulin replacement therapy has been associated with considerable limitations: (i) the excess glucagon levels cannot be addressed /normalized [75, 76], (ii) the insulin analogs do not mimic the endogenous insulin mode of action totally [77], and (iii) intense insulin use triggers weight gain and obesity which induces considerable cardiovascular risk [78, 79]. In summary, an ideal treatment for T1D should address the abnormal beta-cell function, improve HbA1c levels with minimal GV and risk of hypoglycemia, and induce weight control. To offer comprehensive treatment, a combination of insulin displacement therapy with non-insulin agents such as amylin analogs, glucagon-like-peptide-1 (GLP-1) receptor agonists, sodium-glucose co-transporter 2 inhibitors (SGLT2i), and metformin [75, 80].

Amylin is a hormone, co-secreted with insulin, and has glucoregulatory effects that complement insulin, especially on the glucose distribution to the cells during mealtime. A study from Ratner *et al.* demonstrated that combined one-year-long replacement therapy with amylin and insulin analogs improves long-term glycemic control and weight loss in T1D patients [81]. A more recent study reveals that co-administration of amylin and insulin analogs is far more effective in controlling postprandial glucose levels, and this effect was dose-dependent [82].

Sodium-glucose co-transporters, specifically SGLT-2, selectively localize in the kidney, responsible for the selective adsorption of the hexoses (glucose, galactose, fructose, mannose, and myoinositol) into the cells [83]. SGLT2 inhibitors are widely used in DM treatment for their ability to prevent glucose transport into the cells [84]. On the other hand, SGLT1 is expressed both in the kidney and the gut; thus, SGLT1 [85] and SGLT2 [86, 87] inhibitors selectively decrease glucose transport activity. Inhibition of this process increases renal glucose excretion and reduces gut glucose absorption, leading to reduced plasma glucose concentrations and a reduction in body weight [88, 89].

GLP-1 is an incretin hormone released from the gut in response to food intake and is associated with insulin-glucagon secretion [90] and the protection of pancreatic beta-cells against apoptosis [91]. The beneficial effects of GLP-1 receptor agonists in T2D management are well described. However, further findings are required for T1D [75]. The limited number of studies assessing the safety and the efficacy of GLP-1 receptor agonists adapted within the insulin replacement therapy demonstrates a dose-dependent reduction of HbA1c, insulin dose, and weight loss; however, the reports of symptomatic hypoglycemia and hyperglycemia with ketosis prevent its further use in the clinic [92, 93].

Metformin is a plant-based drug known to have a role in glucose metabolism. Although the exact mechanism of metformin needs further investigation, it acts on hepatic gluconeogenesis and reduces the production of glucose [75, 94]. Studies have yielded inconsistent results regarding glycemia, lipids, weight, and insulin-dose reduction, a meta-analysis noted reductions in weight, insulin-dose requirement, and HbA1c but exhibited increased hypoglycemia [95].

Another recent non-insulin-based treatment is an immunotherapy. Teplizumab is a humanized antibody that targets the ε-chain of CD3 molecule expressed in T cells [96]. The strategy behind this particular immunotherapy is blocking especially CD8+ T cell activity *via* Teplizumab binding. This will alter the T cell activation and delay the T cell-mediated destruction of beta-cells. Both Herold *et al.* [97] and Sims *et al.* [98] demonstrated that Teplizumab treatment induces exhausted CD8+ T cells, which are unable to attack the pancreatic beta-cells confirmed by the C-peptide levels. Additionally, significant restoration of insulin levels and reduced autoimmunity were confirmed by the decline of autoreactive CD8+ T cells and TNF-α IFN-γ levels after Teplizumab treatment [98].

3.4 Surgical treatment for T1DM

The treatment approaches for T1D are imperfect, and long-term use of insulin replacement therapy with poor glycemic control leads to systemic complications such as retinopathy, neuropathy, and vasculopathy [99]. The mortality in T1D patients who are younger than 30 years old is due to acute complications, acute ketoacidosis, and hypoglycemia, whereas older patients suffer from cardiovascular disease [100]. Current technologies offer whole organ pancreas or pancreatic islet transplantation as the only options for normal beta-cell replacement to prevent hypoglycemia effectively, restore normoglycemia, and stabilize even prevent complications of T1D [101]. Since the surgical is transplantation, further use of immunosuppressives is crucial for the viability of the transplant. There are three main options regarding pancreas transplantation procedures depending on the patient's kidney function status: (i) pancreas transplant alone (PTA), (ii) pancreas after kidney transplantation (PAK), and (iii) simultaneous pancreas-kidney transplantation (SPK) [102]. SPK transplantation is a gold standard for patients who have pre- or end-stage renal disease [99] and compromises 70% of T1D patients [103]. Nevertheless, PAK transplantations are implemented in 20% of T1D patients who either have a well-functioning living kidney or where the previous SPK has failed [102, 103]. Whole organ pancreas transplantation is restricted to T1D patients without renal impairment, who are unresponsive to available therapies such as insulin replacement, experience frequent and severe hypoglycemia, and poor glycemic control [101]. PTA is an uncommonly performed procedure in 10% of patients [103] and is mainly restricted to younger non-obese patients [99, 101]. Long-term survival of patients who underwent any form of pancreas transplantation showed a significantly improved survival during the 10 years of follow-up period: 70% for SPK and PAK, and 80% for PTA [104]. Ten-year graft survival was 60% for SPK and 40% for the PTA transplantation group [104].

Islet transplantation (IT) is a procedure where pancreatic islet from the patient (autologous) or from a deceased donor (allogenic) is collected, isolated, and transplanted to the patient intraportally via the splenic vein stump, a mesenteric vein, or recannulation of the umbilical vein [105]. Autologous islet transplantation is associated with increased complications because of pancreas resection and transplantation of islets from a diseased pancreas, lowering the success of the treatment [105]. On the other hand, islet allotransplantation is less invasive and has better outcomes, so allo-islet transplantation is considered an alternative, complementary procedure for whole pancreas transplantation [105]. Although allo-islet transplantation is challenging due to the requirement of a compatible donor, advancements in newer stem cell therapies and pancreatic beta-cell substitutes show promising results in preclinical models [106, 107]. IT was classified as an experimental procedure by the American Diabetes Association; thus, data regarding efficacy and safety is limited compared to traditional pancreas transplantation procedures [100]. Nevertheless, islet transplantation alone (ITA) is linked with less technical complications but reduced frequency of insulin-independence compared to PTA [100].

Clinical trials concerning the long-term effects of SPK/SIK and PAK/IAK transplantation presented sustained improvement of glycemic control with slightly elevated HbA1c levels in the PAK/IAK group with a follow-up period of 13 years [108]. Islet transplantation is also performed with a lower risk of complications compared to whole pancreas transplants [108].

4. Conclusion

In conclusion, T1D remains a challenging chronic condition, with 12 million suffer from it. Current technologies are imperfect, and better devices and delivery systems with more accurate and multifunctional abilities are required. Advancements in management techniques, glucose monitoring technologies, and insulin therapies have significantly improved glycemic control and HbA1c levels and reduced GV and patient outcomes. The evolution of commercial insulin products, from rapid-acting and long-acting analogs, offered personalized management regimens for the patients. Additionally, the delivery systems and adjunct therapies to balance the gluconeogenesis cycle are promising emerging approaches to improve patient life quality.

The delivery *via* CSII and hybrid closed-loop systems has enhanced glucose control and reduced the need for MDIs. Insulin delivery systems such as artificial pancreatic systems have revolutionized glucose-level tracking and automated both basal and bolus insulin delivery, enabling more precise and personalized treatment plans with a prospective success rate. Globally, modern delivery devices offer more consistent and controlled insulin administration, improving glycemic outcomes and reducing hypoglycemia risks. Additionally, surgical-based therapies, including pancreas and islet cell transplantation, are the only intervention that provides the potential for long-term remission by restoring pancreatic beta-cell function. However, transplantation comes with significant risks and is not universally applicable. The integration of non-insulin adjuvant therapies provides additional benefits, offering a comprehensive approach to T1D management. However, more immunotherapies such as Teplizumab administration would be beneficial to eliminate insulin deficiency and restore beta-cell function. Immunotherapy approaches provide a treatment with minimal to no complications whether coming from the surgery or the long-term use of exogenous insulin and GV.

Author details

Muzaffer Serdar Deniz
Department of Endocrinology, Sincan Education and Research Hospital, Ankara, Turkey

*Address all correspondence to: md.mserdardeniz@gmail.com

References

[1] Mayer-Davis EJ, Kahkoska AR, Jefferies C, Dabelea D, Balde N, et al. ISPAD clinical practice consensus guidelines 2018: Definition, epidemiology, and classification of diabetes in children and adolescents. Pediatric Diabetes. 2018;**19**:7-19. DOI: 10.1111/pedi.12773

[2] Vollset SE, Ababneh HS, Abate YH, Abbafati C, Abbasgholizadeh R, et al. Burden of disease scenarios for 204 countries and territories, 2022-2050: A forecasting analysis for the global burden of disease study 2021. Lancet. 2024;**403**(10440):2204-2256. DOI: 10.1016/S0140-6736(24)00685-8

[3] Gregory GA, Robinson TIG, Linklater SE, Wang F, Colagiuri S, et al. Global incidence, prevalence, and mortality of type 1 diabetes in 2021 with projection to 2040: A modelling study. The Lancet Diabetes and Endocrinology. 2022;**10**:741-760. DOI: 10.1016/S2213-8587(22)00218-2

[4] Norris JM, Johnson RK, Stene LC. Type 1 diabetes—Early life origins and changing epidemiology. The Lancet Diabetes and Endocrinology. 2020;**8**(3):226-238. DOI: 10.1016/S2213-8587(19)30412-7

[5] Ruiz-Grao MC, Díez-Fernández A, Mesas AE, Martínez-Vizcaíno V, Sequí-Domínguez I, et al. Trends in the incidence of type 1 diabetes in European children and adolescents from 1994 to 2022: A systematic review and meta-analysis. Pediatric Diabetes. 2024;**2024**:1-13. DOI: 10.1155/2024/2338922

[6] Zajec A, Trebušak Podkrajšek K, Tesovnik T, Šket R, Čugalj Kern B, et al. Pathogenesis of type 1 diabetes: Established facts and new insights. Genes (Basel). 2022;**13**(4):706. DOI: 10.3390/genes13040706

[7] Paschou SA, Papadopoulou-Marketou N, Chrousos GP, Kanaka-Gantenbein C. On type 1 diabetes mellitus pathogenesis. Endocrine Connections. 2018;**7**(1):R38-R46. DOI: 10.1530/EC-17-0347

[8] Zorena K, Michalska M, Kurpas M, Jaskulak M, Murawska A, et al. Environmental factors and the risk of developing type 1 diabetes—Old disease and new data. Biology (Basel). 2022;**11**(4):608. DOI: 10.3390/biology11040608

[9] Chiou J, Geusz RJ, Okino ML, Han JY, Miller M, et al. Interpreting type 1 diabetes risk with genetics and single-cell epigenomics. Nature. 2021;**594**(7863):398-402. DOI: 10.1038/s41586-021-03552-w

[10] Redondo MJ, Gignoux CR, Dabelea D, Hagopian WA, Onengut-Gumuscu S, et al. Type 1 diabetes in diverse ancestries and the use of genetic risk scores. The Lancet Diabetes and Endocrinology. 2022;**10**(8):597-608. DOI: 10.1016/S2213-8587(22)00159-0

[11] Howson JMM, Stevens H, Smyth DJ, Walker NM, Chandler KA, et al. Evidence that HLA class I and II associations with type 1 diabetes, autoantibodies to GAD and autoantibodies to IA-2, are distinct. Diabetes. 2011;**60**(10):2635-2644. DOI: 10.2337/db11-0131

[12] Chiang JL, Maahs DM, Garvey KC, Hood KK, Laffel LM, et al. Type 1 diabetes in children and adolescents: A position statement by the American Diabetes Association. Diabetes Care.

2018;**41**(9):2026-2044. DOI: 10.2337/dci18-0023

[13] Janež A, Guja C, Mitrakou A, Lalic N, Tankova T, et al. Insulin therapy in adults with type 1 diabetes mellitus: A narrative review. Diabetes Therapy. 2020;**11**(2):387-409. DOI: 10.1007/s13300-019-00743-7

[14] ElSayed NA, Aleppo G, Aroda VR, Bannuru RR, Brown FM, et al. 14. Children and adolescents: Standards of Care in Diabetes—2023. Diabetes Care. 2023;**46**(Supplement. 1):S230-S253. DOI: 10.2337/dc23-S014

[15] Weinstock R, Aleppo G, Bailey T, Bergenstal R, Fisher W, et al. The role of blood glucose monitoring in diabetes management. ADA Clinical Compendia. 2020;**2020**(3):1-32. DOI: 10.2337/db2020-31

[16] Chehregosha H, Khamseh ME, Malek M, Hosseinpanah F, Ismail-Beigi F. A view beyond HbA1c: Role of continuous glucose monitoring. Diabetes Therapy. 2019;**10**(3):853-863. DOI: 10.1007/s13300-019-0619-1

[17] Cardona-Hernandez R, Dôvc K, Biester T, Ekhlaspour L, Macedoni M, et al. New therapies towards a better glycemic control in youths with type 1 diabetes. Pharmacological Research. 2023;**195**:106882. DOI: 10.1016/j.phrs.2023.106882

[18] Mathew TK, Zubair M, Tadi P, Hospital I, Network H. Blood Glucose Monitoring Pathophysiology. Treasure Island (FL): StatPearls Publishing; 2024. pp. 1-11

[19] Villena Gonzales W, Mobashsher A, Abbosh A. The Progress of glucose monitoring—A review of invasive to minimally and non-invasive techniques, devices and sensors. Sensors. 2019;**19**(4):800. DOI: 10.3390/s19040800

[20] Sia HK, Kor CT, Tu ST, Liao PY, Wang JY. Self-monitoring of blood glucose in association with glycemic control in newly diagnosed non-insulin-treated diabetes patients: A retrospective cohort study. Scientific Reports. 2021;**11**(1):1176. DOI: 10.1038/s41598-021-81024-x

[21] Babaya N, Noso S, Hiromine Y, Taketomo Y, Niwano F, et al. Flash glucose monitoring in type 1 diabetes: A comparison with self-monitoring blood glucose. Journal of Diabetes Investigation. 2020;**11**(5):1222-1229. DOI: 10.1111/jdi.13229

[22] Kumar Das S, Nayak KK, Krishnaswamy PR, Kumar V, Bhat N. Review—Electrochemistry and other emerging technologies for continuous glucose monitoring devices. ECS Sensors Plus. 2022;**1**(3):031601. DOI: 10.1149/2754-2726/ac7abb

[23] Karter AJ, Parker MM, Moffet HH, Gilliam LK, Dlott R. Association of real-time continuous glucose monitoring with glycemic control and acute metabolic events among patients with insulin-treated diabetes. JAMA. 2021;**325**(22):2273. DOI: 10.1001/jama.2021.6530

[24] Edelman SV, Argento NB, Pettus J, Hirsch IB. Clinical implications of real-time and intermittently scanned continuous glucose monitoring. Diabetes Care. 2018;**41**(11):2265-2274. DOI: 10.2337/dc18-1150

[25] Di Molfetta S, Caruso I, Cignarelli A, Natalicchio A, Perrini S, et al. Professional continuous glucose monitoring in patients with diabetes mellitus: A systematic review and meta-analysis. Diabetes, Obesity and Metabolism. 2023;**25**(5):1301-1310. DOI: 10.1111/dom.14981

[26] Maiorino MI, Signoriello S, Maio A, Chiodini P, Bellastella G, et al. Effects of continuous glucose monitoring on metrics of glycemic control in diabetes: A systematic review with meta-analysis of randomized controlled trials. Diabetes Care. 2020;**43**(5):1146-1156. DOI: 10.2337/dc19-1459

[27] Wada E, Onoue T, Kobayashi T, Handa T, Hayase A, et al. Flash glucose monitoring helps achieve better glycemic control than conventional self-monitoring of blood glucose in non-insulin-treated type 2 diabetes: A randomized controlled trial. BMJ Open Diabetes Research & Care. 2020;**8**(1):e001115. DOI: 10.1136/bmjdrc-2019-001115

[28] Hásková A, Radovnická L, Petruželková L, Parkin CG, Grunberger G, et al. Real-time CGM is superior to flash glucose monitoring for glucose control in type 1 diabetes: The CORRIDA randomized controlled trial. Diabetes Care. 2020;**43**(11):2744-2750. DOI: 10.2337/dc20-0112

[29] Pleus S, Ulbrich S, Zschornack E, Kamann S, Haug C, et al. Documentation of skin-related issues associated with continuous glucose monitoring use in the scientific literature. Diabetes Technology & Therapeutics. 2019;**21**(10):538-545. DOI: 10.1089/dia.2019.0171

[30] Asarani NAM, Reynolds AN, Boucher SE, de Bock M, Wheeler BJ. Cutaneous complications with continuous or flash glucose monitoring use: Systematic review of trials and observational studies. Journal of Diabetes Science and Technology. 2020;**14**(2):328-337. DOI: 10.1177/1932296819870849

[31] Hyry HSI, Liippo JP, Virtanen HM. Allergic contact dermatitis caused by glucose sensors in type 1 diabetes patients. Contact Dermatitis. 2019;**81**(3):161-166. DOI: 10.1111/cod.13337

[32] Battelino T, Danne T, Bergenstal RM, Amiel SA, Beck R, et al. Clinical targets for continuous glucose monitoring data interpretation: Recommendations from the international consensus on time in range. Diabetes Care. 2019;**42**(8):1593-1603. DOI: 10.2337/dci19-0028

[33] Dovc K, Battelino T. Time in range centered diabetes care. Clinical Pediatric Endocrinology. 2021;**30**(1):1-10. DOI: 10.1297/cpe.30.1

[34] Sanchez P, Ghosh-Dastidar S, Tweden KS, Kaufman FR. Real-world data from the first U.S. commercial users of an implantable continuous glucose sensor. Diabetes Technology & Therapeutics. 2019;**21**(12):677-681. DOI: 10.1089/dia.2019.0234

[35] Rydén L, Lindsten J. The history of the Nobel prize for the discovery of insulin. Diabetes Research and Clinical Practice. 2021;**175**:108819. DOI: 10.1016/j.diabres.2021.108819

[36] Sims EK, Carr ALJ, Oram RA, DiMeglio LA, Evans-Molina C. 100 years of insulin: Celebrating the past, present and future of diabetes therapy. Nature Medicine. 2021;**27**(7):1154-1164. DOI: 10.1038/s41591-021-01418-2

[37] Eliaschewitz FG, Barreto T. Concepts and clinical use of ultra-long basal insulin. Diabetology and Metabolic Syndrome. 2016;**8**(1):2. DOI: 10.1186/s13098-015-0117-1

[38] Ovalle F, Segal AR, Anderson JE, Cohen MR, Morwick TM, et al. Understanding concentrated insulins: A systematic review of randomized controlled trials. Current Medical Research and Opinion. 2018;**34**(6):1029-1043. DOI: 10.1080/03007995.2017.1409426

[39] Sundberg F, DeBeaufort C, Krogvold L, Patton S, Piloya T, et al. ISPAD clinical practice consensus guidelines 2022: Managing diabetes in preschoolers. Pediatric Diabetes. 2022;**23**(8):1496-1511. DOI: 10.1111/pedi.13427

[40] Giorgino F, Battelino T, Bergenstal RM, Forst T, Green JB, et al. The role of ultra-rapid-acting insulin analogs in diabetes: An expert consensus. Journal of Diabetes Science and Technology. 2023:19322968231204584. DOI: 10.1177/19322968231204584

[41] Wong EY, Kroon L. Ultra-rapid-acting insulins: How fast is really needed? Clinical Diabetes. 2021;**39**(4):415-423. DOI: 10.2337/cd20-0119

[42] Kildegaard J, Buckley ST, Nielsen RH, Povlsen GK, Seested T, et al. Elucidating the mechanism of absorption of fast-acting insulin aspart: The role of niacinamide. Pharmaceutical Research. 2019;**36**(3):1-14. DOI: 10.1007/s11095-019-2578-7

[43] Olsen HB, Havelund S, Ribel-Madsen U, Sturis J, Naver H, et al. United States Patent. US Patent; US 8. 2012;**2**:(12):324,157 B2,

[44] Kazda C, Leohr J, Liu R, Reddy S, Dellva MA, et al. Ultra rapid lispro (URLi) shows accelerated pharmacokinetics and greater reduction in postprandial glucose versus Humalog® in patients with type 1 diabetes mellitus in a randomized, double-blind meal test early-phase study. Diabetes, Obesity and Metabolism. 2022;**24**(2):196-203. DOI: 10.1111/dom.14563

[45] Leohr J, Dellva MA, Carter K, LaBell E, Linnebjerg H. Ultra rapid lispro (URLi) accelerates insulin lispro absorption and insulin action vs Humalog® consistently across study populations: A pooled analysis of pharmacokinetic and glucodynamic data. Clinical Pharmacokinetics. 2021;**60**(11):1423-1434. DOI: 10.1007/s40262-021-01030-0

[46] Malecki MT, Cao D, Liu R, Hardy T, Bode B, et al. Ultra-rapid lispro improves postprandial glucose control and time in range in type 1 diabetes compared to lispro: PRONTO-T1D continuous glucose monitoring substudy. Diabetes Technology & Therapeutics. 2020;**22**(11):853-860. DOI: 10.1089/dia.2020.0129

[47] Klaff L, Cao D, Dellva MA, Tobian J, Miura J, et al. Ultra rapid lispro improves postprandial glucose control compared with lispro in patients with type 1 diabetes: Results from the 26-week PRONTO-T1D study. Diabetes, Obesity and Metabolism. 2020;**22**(10):1799-1807. DOI: 10.1111/dom.14100

[48] Zhou J, Chen S, Cheng J, Zhu J, Lou Y, et al. Ultra rapid lispro improves postprandial glucose control versus lispro in combination with insulin glargine/degludec in adults with type 2 diabetes: A prospective, randomized, double-blind, phase 3 trial. Scientific Bulletin. 2022;**67**(17):1785-1791. DOI: 10.1016/j.scib.2022.08.002

[49] Pieber TR, Eugene-Jolchine I, Derobert E. Efficacy and safety of HOE 901 versus NPH insulin in patients with type 1 diabetes. Diabetes Care. 2000;**23**(2):157-162

[50] Saboo B, Chandalia H, Ghosh S, Kesavadev J, Kochar I, et al. Insulin glargine in type 1 diabetes mellitus: A review of clinical trials and real-world evidence across two decades. Current Diabetes Reviews. 2024;**20**(1):27-41. DOI: 10.2174/1573399819666230310150905

[51] Matsuhisa M, Koyama M, Cheng X, Takahashi Y, Riddle MC, et al. New insulin glargine 300 U/ml versus glargine 100 U/ml in Japanese adults with type 1 diabetes using basal and mealtime insulin: Glucose control and hypoglycaemia in a randomized controlled trial (EDITION JP 1). Diabetes, Obesity and Metabolism. 2016;**18**(4):375-383. DOI: 10.1111/dom.12619

[52] Joshi SR, Singh G, Marwah A, Mittra S, Suvarna VR, et al. Comparative clinical efficacy and safety of insulin glargine 300 U/ml (Toujeo) versus insulin glargine 100 U/ml in type 2 diabetes and type 1 diabetes: A systematic literature review and meta-analysis. Diabetes, Obesity and Metabolism. 2023;**25**(6):1589-1606. DOI: 10.1111/dom.15007

[53] Danne T, Tamborlane WV, Malievsky OA, Franco DR, Kawamura T, et al. Efficacy and safety of insulin glargine 300 units/mL (Gla-300) versus insulin glargine 100 units/mL (Gla-100) in children and adolescents (6-17 years) with type 1 diabetes: Results of the EDITION JUNIOR randomized controlled trial. Diabetes Care. 2020;**43**(7):1512-1519. DOI: 10.2337/dc19-1926

[54] Home P, Kurtzhals P. Insulin detemir: From concept to clinical experience. Expert Opinion on Pharmacotherapy. 2006;7(3):325-343. DOI: 10.1517/14656566.7.3.325

[55] Vora J, Cariou B, Evans M, Gross JL, Harris S, et al. Clinical use of insulin degludec. Diabetes Research and Clinical Practice. 2015;**109**(1):19-31. DOI: 10.1016/j.diabres.2015.04.002

[56] Alhmoud EN, Saad MO, Omar NE. Efficacy and safety of insulin glargine 300 units/mL vs insulin degludec in patients with type 1 and type 2 diabetes: A systematic review and meta-analysis. Front Endocrinol (Lausanne). 2024;**14**(January):1-13. DOI: 10.3389/fendo.2023.1285147

[57] Gomez-Peralta F, Chico Ballesteros A, Marco Martínez A, Pérez Corral B, Conget Donlo I, et al. Insulin glargine 300 U/ ml versus insulin degludec 100 U/ ml improves nocturnal glycaemic control and variability in type 1 diabetes under routine clinical practice: A glucodensities-based post hoc analysis of the OneCare study. Diabetes, Obesity and Metabolism. 2024;**26**(5):1993-1997. DOI: 10.1111/dom.15496

[58] Pozzilli P, Battelino T, Danne T, Hovorka R, Jarosz-Chobot P, et al. Continuous subcutaneous insulin infusion in diabetes: Patient populations, safety, efficacy, and pharmacoeconomics. Diabetes/Metabolism Research and Reviews. 2016;**32**(1):21-39. DOI: 10.1002/dmrr.2653

[59] Tauschmann M, Hovorka R. Technology in the management of type 1 diabetes mellitus—Current status and future prospects. Nature Reviews. Endocrinology. 2018;**14**(8):464-475. DOI: 10.1038/s41574-018-0044-y

[60] Sherr JL, Hermann JM, Campbell F, Foster NC, Hofer SE, et al. Use of insulin pump therapy in children and adolescents with type 1 diabetes and its impact on metabolic control: Comparison of results from three large, transatlantic paediatric registries. Diabetologia. 2016;**59**(1):87-91. DOI: 10.1007/s00125-015-3790-6

[61] Karges B, Schwandt A, Heidtmann B, Kordonouri O, Binder E, et al. Association of insulin pump therapy vs insulin injection therapy with severe hypoglycemia, ketoacidosis,

and glycemic control among children, adolescents, and young adults with type 1 diabetes. JAMA. 2017;**318**(14):1358-1366. DOI: 10.1001/jama.2017.13994

[62] Little SA, Leelarathna L, Walkinshaw E, Tan HK, Chapple O, et al. Recovery of hypoglycemia awareness in long-standing type 1 diabetes: A multicenter 2 × 2 factorial randomized controlled trial comparing insulin pump with multiple daily injections and continuous with conventional glucose self-monitoring (HypoCOMPaSS). Diabetes Care. 2014;**37**(8):2114-2122. DOI: 10.2337/dc14-0030

[63] Moon SJ, Jung I, Park CY. Current advances of artificial pancreas systems: A comprehensive review of the clinical evidence. Diabetes and Metabolism Journal. 2021;**45**(6):813-839. DOI: 10.4093/dmj.2021.0177

[64] Kulzer B, Freckmann G, Heinemann L, Schnell O, Hinzmann R, et al. Patch pumps: What are the advantages for people with diabetes? Diabetes Research and Clinical Practice. 2022;**187**(April):109858. DOI: 10.1016/j.diabres.2022.109858

[65] Templer S. Closed-loop insulin delivery systems: Past, present, and future directions. Front Endocrinol (Lausanne). 2022;**13**(June):1-9. DOI: 10.3389/fendo.2022.919942

[66] Bergenstal RM, Tamborlane WV, Ahmann A, Buse JB, Dailey G, et al. Sensor-augmented pump therapy for A1C reduction (STAR 3) study. Diabetes Care. 2011;**34**(11):2403-2405. DOI: 10.2337/dc11-1248

[67] Hermanides J, Nørgaard K, Bruttomesso D, Mathieu C, Frid A, et al. Sensor-augmented pump therapy lowers HbA1c in suboptimally controlled type 1 diabetes: A randomized controlled trial. Diabetic Medicine. 2011;**28**(10):1158-1167. DOI: 10.1111/j.1464-5491.2011.03256.x

[68] Hovorka R. Closed-loop insulin delivery: From bench to clinical practice. Nature Reviews. Endocrinology. 2011;**7**(7):385-395. DOI: 10.1038/nrendo.2011.32

[69] Bergenstal RM, Garg S, Weinzimer SA, Buckingham BA, Bode BW, et al. Safety of a hybrid closed-loop insulin delivery system in patients with type 1 diabetes. Journal of the American Medical Association. 2016;**316**(13):1407. DOI: 10.1001/jama.2016.11708

[70] Garg SK, Weinzimer SA, Tamborlane WV, Buckingham BA, Bode BW, et al. Glucose outcomes with the In-Home use of a hybrid closed-loop insulin delivery system in adolescents and adults with type 1 diabetes. Diabetes Technology & Therapeutics. 2017;**19**(3):155-163. DOI: 10.1089/dia.2016.0421

[71] Sherr JL, Heinemann L, Fleming GA, Bergenstal RM, Bruttomesso D, et al. Automated insulin delivery: Benefits, challenges, and recommendations. A consensus report of the joint diabetes technology working Group of the European Association for the study of diabetes and the American Diabetes Association. Diabetologia. 2023;**66**(1):3-22. DOI: 10.1007/s00125-022-05744-z

[72] Quattrin T, Mastrandrea LD, Walker LSK. Type 1 diabetes. Lancet. 2023;**401**(10394):2149-2162. DOI: 10.1016/S0140-6736(23)00223-4

[73] Russell SJ, El-Khatib FH, Sinha M, Magyar KL, McKeon K, et al. Outpatient glycemic control with a bionic pancreas in type 1 diabetes. The New England Journal of Medicine. 2014;**371**(4):313-325. DOI: 10.1056/NEJMoa1314474

[74] Bionic Pancreas Research Group. Multicenter, randomized trial of a bionic pancreas in type 1 diabetes. The New England Journal of Medicine. 2022;**387**(13):1161-1172. DOI: 10.1056/nejmoa2205225

[75] Frandsen CS, Dejgaard TF, Madsbad S. Non-insulin drugs to treat hyperglycaemia in type 1 diabetes mellitus. The Lancet Diabetes and Endocrinology. 2016;**4**(9):766-780. DOI: 10.1016/S2213-8587(16)00039-5

[76] Snaith JR, Holmes-Walker DJ, Greenfield JR. Reducing type 1 diabetes mortality: Role for adjunctive therapies? Trends in Endocrinology and Metabolism. 2020;**31**(2):150-164. DOI: 10.1016/j.tem.2019.11.007

[77] Woerle HJ, Albrecht M, Linke R, Zschau S, Neumann C, et al. Impaired hyperglycemia-induced delay in gastric emptying in patients with type 1 diabetes deficient for islet amyloid polypeptide. Diabetes Care. 2008;**31**(12):2325-2331. DOI: 10.2337/dc07-2446

[78] Kilpatrick ES, Rigby AS, Atkin SL. Insulin resistance, the metabolic syndrome, and complication risk in type 1 diabetes. Diabetes Care. 2007;**30**(3):707-712. DOI: 10.2337/dc06-1982

[79] Conway B, Miller RG, Costacou T, Fried L, Kelsey S, et al. Temporal patterns in overweight and obesity in type 1 diabetes. Diabetic Medicine. 2010;**27**(4):398-404. DOI: 10.1111/j.1464-5491.2010.02956.x

[80] Galindo RJ, Dhatariya K, Gomez-Peralta F, Umpierrez GE. Safety and efficacy of inpatient diabetes management with non-insulin agents: An overview of international practices. Current Diabetes Reports. 2022;**22**(6):237-246. DOI: 10.1007/s11892-022-01464-1

[81] Ratner RE, Dickey R, Fineman M, Maggs DG, Shen L, et al. Amylin replacement with pramlintide as an adjunct to insulin therapy improves long-term glycaemic and weight control in type 1 diabetes mellitus: A 1-year, randomized controlled trial. Diabetic Medicine. 2004;**21**(11):1204-1212. DOI: 10.1111/j.1464-5491.2004.01319.x

[82] Riddle MC, Yuen KCJ, de Bruin TW, Herrmann K, Xu J, et al. Fixed ratio dosing of pramlintide with regular insulin before a standard meal in patients with type 1 diabetes. Diabetes, Obesity and Metabolism. 2015;**17**(9):904-907. DOI: 10.1111/dom.12504

[83] Ferrannini E. Sodium-glucose co-transporters and their inhibition: Clinical physiology. Cell Metabolism. 2017;**26**(1):27-38. DOI: 10.1016/j.cmet.2017.04.011

[84] Nespoux J, Vallon V. SGLT2 inhibition and kidney protection. Clinical Science. 2018;**132**(12):1329-1339. DOI: 10.1042/CS20171298

[85] Song P, Onishi A, Koepsell H, Vallon V. Sodium glucose co-transporter SGLT1 as a therapeutic target in diabetes mellitus. Expert Opinion on Therapeutic Targets. 2016;**20**(9):1109-1125. DOI: 10.1517/14728222.2016.1168808

[86] Rosenstock J, Marquard J, Laffel LM, Neubacher D, Kaspers S, et al. Empagliflozin as adjunctive to insulin therapy in type 1 diabetes: The EASE trials. Diabetes Care. 2018;**41**(12):2560-2569. DOI: 10.2337/dc18-1749

[87] Dandona P, Mathieu C, Phillip M, Hansen L, Griffen SC, et al. Efficacy and safety of dapagliflozin in patients with inadequately controlled type 1 diabetes (DEPICT-1): 24 week results from a multicentre, double-blind, phase 3, randomised controlled trial. The

Lancet Diabetes and Endocrinology. 2017;**5**(11):864-876. DOI: 10.1016/S2213-8587(17)30308-X

[88] Sands AT, Zambrowicz BP, Rosenstock J, Lapuerta P, Bode BW, et al. Sotagliflozin, a dual SGLT1 and SGLT2 inhibitor, as adjunct therapy to insulin in type 1 diabetes. Diabetes Care. 2015;**38**(7):1181-1188. DOI: 10.2337/dc14-2806

[89] Garg SK, Henry RR, Banks P, Buse JB, Davies MJ, et al. Effects of sotagliflozin added to insulin in patients with type 1 diabetes. The New England Journal of Medicine. 2017;**377**(24):2337-2348. DOI: 10.1056/NEJMoa1708337

[90] Kaneto H, Kimura T, Shimoda M, Obata A, Sanada J, et al. Favorable effects of GLP-1 receptor agonist against pancreatic β-cell glucose toxicity and the development of arteriosclerosis: "The earlier, the better" in therapy with incretin-based medicine. International Journal of Molecular Sciences. 2021;**22**(15):7917. DOI: 10.3390/ijms22157917

[91] Chang TJ, Tseng HC, Liu MW, Chang YC, Hsieh ML, et al. Glucagon-like peptide-1 prevents methylglyoxal-induced apoptosis of beta cells through improving mitochondrial function and suppressing prolonged AMPK activation. Scientific Reports. 2016;**6**:23403. DOI: 10.1038/srep23403

[92] Ahrén B, Hirsch IB, Pieber TR, Mathieu C, Gómez-Peralta F, et al. Efficacy and safety of liraglutide added to capped insulin treatment in subjects with type 1 diabetes: The ADJUNCT TWO randomized trial. Diabetes Care. 2016;**39**(10):1693-1701. DOI: 10.2337/dc16-0690

[93] Mathieu C, Zinman B, Hemmingsson JU, Woo V, Colman P, et al. Efficacy and safety of liraglutide added to insulin treatment in type 1 diabetes: The ADJUNCT ONE treat-to-target randomized trial. Diabetes Care. 2016;**39**(10):1702-1710. DOI: 10.2337/dc16-0691

[94] Rena G, Hardie DG, Pearson ER. The mechanisms of action of metformin. Diabetologia. 2017;**60**(9):1577-1585. DOI: 10.1007/s00125-017-4342-z

[95] Vella S, Buetow L, Royle P, Livingstone S, Colhoun HM, et al. The use of metformin in type 1 diabetes: A systematic review of efficacy. Diabetologia. 2010;**53**(5):809-820. DOI: 10.1007/s00125-009-1636-9

[96] Herold KC, Bundy BN, Long SA, Bluestone JA, DiMeglio LA, et al. An anti-CD3 antibody, teplizumab, in relatives at risk for type 1 diabetes. The New England Journal of Medicine. 2019;**381**(7):603-613. DOI: 10.1056/NEJMoa1902226

[97] Herold KC, Gitelman SE, Gottlieb PA, Knecht LA, Raymond R, et al. Teplizumab: A disease-modifying therapy for type 1 diabetes that preserves β-cell function. Diabetes Care. 2023;**46**(10):1848-1856. DOI: 10.2337/dc23-0675

[98] Sims EK, Bundy BN, Stier K, Serti E, Lim N, et al. Teplizumab improves and stabilizes beta cell function in antibody-positive high-risk individuals. Science Translational Medicine. 2021;**13**(583):1-14. DOI: 10.1126/scitranslmed.abc8980

[99] Holt RIG, DeVries JH, Hess-Fischl A, Hirsch IB, Kirkman MS, et al. The Management of Type 1 diabetes in adults. A consensus report by the American Diabetes Association (ADA) and the European Association for the Study of diabetes (EASD). Diabetes Care. 2021;**44**(11):2589-2625. DOI: 10.2337/dci21-0043

[100] Maffi P, Secchi A. Islet transplantation alone versus solitary pancreas transplantation: An outcome-driven choice? Current Diabetes Reports. 2019;**19**(5):26. DOI: 10.1007/s11892-019-1145-2

[101] Piemonti L, Socci C, Nano R, Maffi P, Secchi A. Islet cell or pancreas transplantation. In: Endocrinology (Switzerland). Cham: Springer; 2018. pp. 655-693. DOI: 10.1007/978-3-319-45015-5_23

[102] Lerner SM. Kidney and pancreas transplantation in type 1 diabetes mellitus. Mount Sinai Journal of Medicine A J Transl Personalized Medicine. 2008;**75**(4):372-384. DOI: 10.1002/msj.20056

[103] Kochar IS, Jain R. Pancreas transplant in type 1 diabetes mellitus: The emerging role of islet cell transplant. Annals of Pediatric Endocrinology & Metabolism. 2021;**26**(2):86-91. DOI: 10.6065/apem.2142012.006

[104] Gruessner AC, Gruessner RWG. Long-term outcome after pancreas transplantation. Current Opinion in Organ Transplantation. 2016;**21**(4):377-385. DOI: 10.1097/MOT.0000000000000331

[105] Rickels MR, Robertson RP. Pancreatic islet transplantation in humans: Recent Progress and future directions. Endocrine Reviews. 2019;**40**(2):631-668. DOI: 10.1210/er.2018-00154

[106] Yang L, Hu ZM, Jiang FX, Wang W. Stem cell therapy for insulin-dependent diabetes: Are we still on the road? World Journal of Stem Cells. 2022;**14**(7):503-512. DOI: 10.4252/wjsc.v14.i7.503

[107] Parums DV. Editorial: First regulatory approval for allogeneic pancreatic islet Beta cell infusion for adult patients with type 1 diabetes mellitus. Medical Science Monitor. 2023;**29**:1-2. DOI: 10.12659/MSM.941918

[108] Lehmann R, Graziano J, Brockmann J, Pfammatter T, Kron P, et al. Glycemic control in simultaneous islet-kidney versus pancreas-kidney transplantation in type 1 diabetes: A prospective 13-year follow-up. Diabetes Care. 2015;**38**(5):752-759. DOI: 10.2337/dc14-1686

Section 3

Care for Complications and Life Quality

Chapter 5

Navigating Life with Type 1 Diabetes: Challenges, Innovations, and Daily Resilience

Yashika Saini, Mohseen and Rajesh Kumar Sharma

Abstract

In this chapter, our focus is to illuminate the multifaceted landscape of type 1 diabetes (T1D), addressing its challenges, innovations, and clinical manifestations. We begin with a thorough overview, delving into the causes and associated risk factors, as well as demographic trends and prevalence figures. We focus on the daily challenges that people with T1D encounter and dive into the complexities of management, emphasising the critical role of insulin therapy. Furthermore, we explore technological developments that have transformed treatment paradigms, providing new perspectives that help in improving quality of life. Keeping up with the most recent research and development developments, we highlight continuing initiatives to improve T1D understanding and treatment options. Finally, we examine the often-overlooked psychosocial aspects of living with this chronic condition, hoping to raise understanding and empathy among healthcare professionals and the general public. This chapter aims to provide new insights into T1D, promoting a nuanced understanding of its complexities and manifestations.

Keywords: type 1 diabetes mellitus, clinical manifestations, insulin therapy, glucose metabolism, innovations in diabetes

1. Introduction

T1D is a chronic, multifactorial, autoimmune disease that is polygenic and marked by the death of pancreatic β-cells, which is linked to long-term dysfunction of multiple organs and tissues [1]. Genetic predisposition, beta cell stressors and their effects, the innate and adaptive immune systems, unclear environmental factors, and other variables all play a role in the pathogenesis of type 1 diabetes. These interactions result in a complex and poorly understood chain of events that starts with normal immune system and beta cell function and progresses to pancreatic beta cell-specific autoimmunity and the eventual clinical manifestation [2]. Significant progress has been made in understanding the mechanisms behind hyperglycemia throughout the past century. An important breakthrough in the understanding of insulin's function in glucose regulation was made in the 1920s by Banting, Best, Collip, and Macleod, who used insulin derived from bovine pancreas to lower a patient's blood glucose levels successfully. Clinical observations started to distinguish between insulin-sensitive and insulin-insensitive forms of diabetes by the middle of the 1930s. The classification of diabetes into "insulin-dependent" (low insulin levels) and "non-insulin-dependent" (normal or high insulin levels) categories occurred in the 1950s as a result of improvements in the measurement of circulating insulin. Additional discoveries in the following decades included the detection of insulin resistance in non-insulin-dependent diabetes and immune-mediated β-cell death in insulin-dependent diabetes. In 1979, the terms "type 1" and "type 2" diabetes were officially recognised. The difference between both types has, however, been less evident in recent years because some individuals show immunological activation against β-cells in addition to insulin resistance. Beyond the conventional glucocentric perspective, advances in cellular and molecular biology point to the possibility of a more complex pathophysiological classification that could enhance patient phenotyping and treatment (**Table 1, Figure 1**) [9].

Basis of differences	Type 1 diabetes	Type 2 diabetes	Reference
1. Onset	It is an autoimmune disease in which pancreatic beta cells that are responsible for producing insulin get damaged.	Adults are more likely to acquire type 2 diabetes (T2D), which is typically brought on by insulin resistance and is frequently linked to obesity and a sedentary lifestyle.	[3, 4]
2. Age	Usually manifests at an earlier age, usually in childhood or adolescence.	Although T2D often first appears in adults, rising childhood incidence is a result of rising obesity rates.	[4, 5]
3. Insulin dependence	Due to insufficient or absence of insulin production by their bodies, people with T1D are dependent on insulin therapy to survive.	On the other hand, many people with T2D may initially be able to control their condition with dietary modifications and oral medications; nevertheless, if the disease worsens, insulin may eventually be required.	[5, 6]
4. Risk factors	Less is known about the risk factors for type 1 diabetes, but these include environmental triggers such as viral infections and genetic predispositions.	Genetic and lifestyle variables, including physical inactivity, poor diet, and obesity, have a substantial impact on type 2 diabetes.	[5]
5. Associated complications	Diabetic ketoacidosis is a prevalent complication among T1D patients, and long-term glycaemic control problems are typically the cause of chronic sequelae such as retinopathy and nephropathy.	Patients with type 2 diabetes frequently experience metabolic syndrome-related side effects, such as neuropathy and cardiovascular illnesses, which are typically linked to obesity and insulin resistance.	[5, 7, 8]
6. Prevalence	T1D is responsible for around 5–10% of all diabetes cases.	However, T2D accounts for 90–95% of all instances of diabetes globally, indicating a higher correlation between age and variables related to lifestyle.	[5]

Table 1.
Difference between type 1 and type 2 diabetes on the basis of different factors.

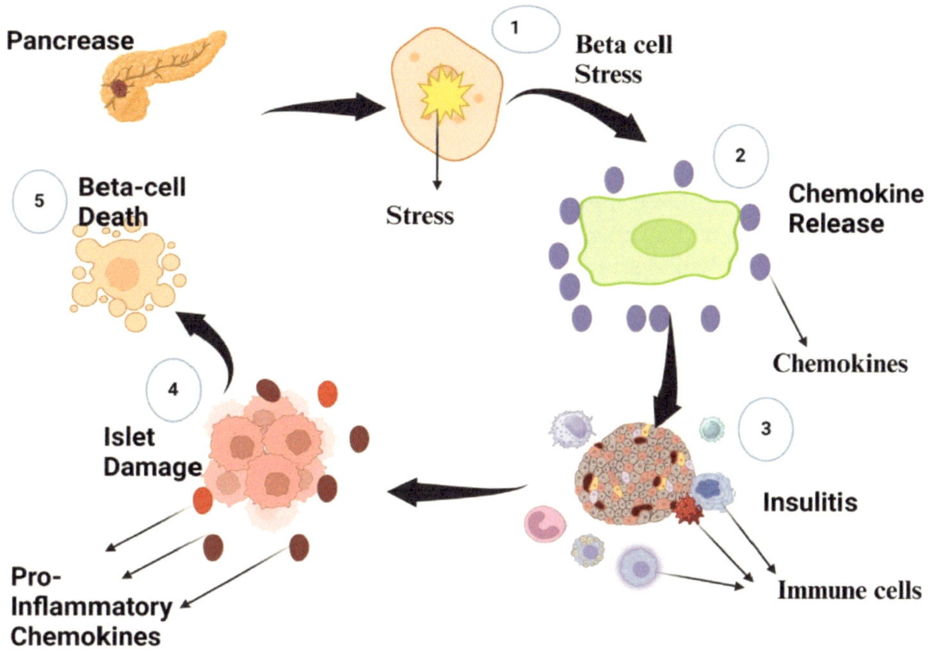

Figure 1.
Stages of type 1 diabetes.

1.1 Understanding the pathophysiology, symptoms, and prevention strategies of hypoglycaemia in type 1 diabetes

As life expectancy increases due to improvements in diabetes care, the number of older adults with type 1 diabetes is growing. Older adults are more likely to experience hypoglycaemia and hypoglycaemia unawareness, especially if they have had type 1 diabetes for a long time. Seizures and falls that result in fractures, cognitive impairment, and cardiac arrhythmias that cause sudden death are all consequences of severe hypoglycaemia, in addition to acute changes in mental status. Treatment recommendations for older adults with type 1 diabetes, therefore, permit less strict haemoglobin A1c (HbA1c) targets and stress-reducing hypoglycaemia by maintaining glucose levels below 70 mg/dL less than 1% of the time. Even so, severe hypoglycaemia is still a frequent side effect [1]. About 30% of people with T1D have severe hypoglycaemia (SH), which is an occurrence that needs outside help and is a significant cause of morbidity [10]. Characteristics of hypoglycaemia in people with type 1 diabetes include confusion, difficulty concentrating, drowsiness, visual disturbances, slurred speech, and dizziness due to neuroglycopenia, as well as symptoms like shakiness, sweating, palpitations, anxiety, and hunger because of autonomic nervous system activation. There may also be general symptoms, including headache, exhaustion, weakness, and irritability. Regular blood glucose checks, adherence to a regular diet and meal plan, modifying insulin dosages in accordance with physical activity levels, and moderation when drinking alcohol are all necessary to prevent hypoglycaemia. The likelihood of severe episodes can be further decreased by providing education on how to identify early symptoms and carry fast-acting glucose, such as glucose tablets or sugary snacks [11].

1.2 Physiological impact on the body

T lymphocyte-mediated insulitis signals the onset of T1D immunologically. This is followed by the existence of one or more forms of autoantibodies that (AAb) against insulin, zinc transporter 8 (ZnT8), glutamic acid decarboxylase (GAD), protein tyrosine phosphatase IA-2 or IA-2β, and insulin [12]. Studies have shown that among young T1D patients, isolated high diastolic blood pressure is more common. Increased diastolic blood pressure has been linked to an imminent risk of hypertension, according to previously published studies. Unhealthy weight increase is a significant risk factor for hypertension, particularly when it involves the buildup of visceral fat. Evidence of the rising incidence and effects of obesity in people with type 1 diabetes is mounting [13]. Patients with type 1 diabetes have increased oxidative stress and

S.No.	Particular	Physiological impairment	Physiological impact	Reference
1	Glucose metabolism	Absolute deficiency of insulin	The liver responds by increasing glucose production	[15, 16]
2	Lipid metabolism	Lack of insulin	Production of ketone bodies, which can lead to diabetic ketoacidosis	[17]
3	Protein metabolism	Lack of insulin	Promotes protein breakdown, muscle wasting, and weight loss	[18, 19]
4	Electrolyte imbalances	Hyperglycemia leads to osmotic diuresis	Significant loss of water and electrolytes, which causes metabolic acidosis	[20]
5	Cardiovascular system	Chronic hyperglycemia, which causes endothelial dysfunction	Increased risk of atherosclerosis and cardiovascular diseases	[21, 22]
6	Nervous system	Prolonged hyperglycemia can lead to diabetic neuropathy	Affecting both peripheral and autonomic nerves, which can result in symptoms like pain, numbness, and organ dysfunction	[23]
7	Renal system	Diabetic nephropathy	Progress to end-stage renal disease, risk of urinary tract infections due to impaired immune function	[24, 25]
8	Ocular system	Diabetic retinopathy	Vision impairment and blindness, cataracts, and glaucoma	[26, 27]
9	Gastrointestinal system	Gastroparesis, autonomic neuropathy	Erratic blood glucose levels and digestive issues	[28, 29]
10	Skeletal system	Chronic hyperglycemia and insulin deficiency	Decreased bone mineral density, increasing the risk of fractures	[30, 31]
11	Immune system	Impairs immune responses	Increasing susceptibility to infections and delaying wound healing	[32, 33]
12	Reproductive system	Chronic hyperglycemia and insulin deficiency	Menstrual irregularities and affect fertility, erectile dysfunction due to vascular and neuropathic complications	[34, 35]

Table 2.
Physiological impairment and impact of T1D.

decreased muscle adenosine triphosphate (ATP) production, which is mostly related to hyperglycemia. Additionally, they could display aberrant liver postprandial glycogen metabolism and fasting [14]. Type 1 diabetes has various physiological impacts on the human body. Here are some physiological impairments and impacts of T1D given in the following **Table 2**.

2. Clinical manifestations and daily challenges

The presence of many AAb types denotes T1D stage 1. Stage 2 is characterised by dysglycemia or glucose intolerance. Stage 3 is marked by the clinical development of symptoms associated with hyperglycemia (enuresis, polyuria, polydipsia, weight loss, blurred vision) and, in certain cases, even diabetic ketoacidosis (DKA) or diabetic hyperosmolar syndrome. The first two stages are asymptomatic [12]. Maintaining overall wellness and health is a key component of managing type 1 diabetes (T1D). Consistent self-care habits are necessary for good diabetes control, according to the U.S. Centres for Disease Control and Prevention (CDCP). These include following a nutritious diet, exercising frequently, and keeping a close eye on blood sugar levels. Even in the absence of symptoms, taking prescribed medications as directed is essential. Essential elements of care also include stress management and emotional support for those with diabetes. Frequent check-ups also contribute to long-term health by assisting people with T1D in incorporating diabetes care into their daily routines (**Figure 2**).

2.1 Managing blood sugar levels

The determination of diabetes is based on three factors: a blood glucose level that is higher than 7·0 mmol/L (126 mg/dL) during fasting, a blood glucose level that is

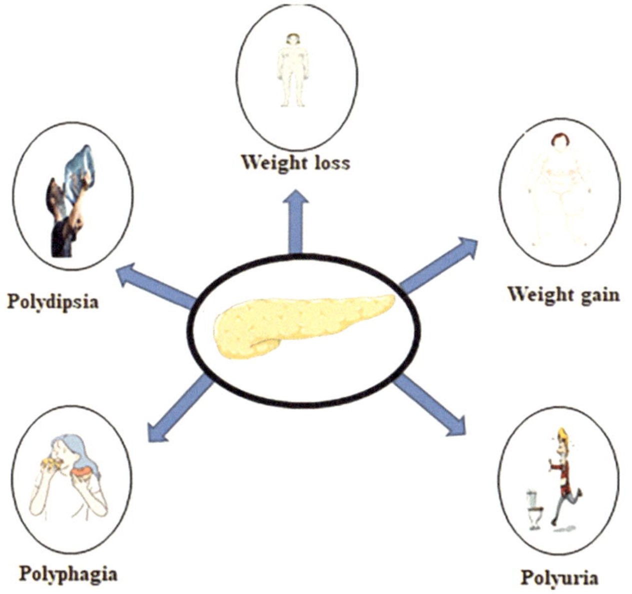

Figure 2.
Clinical manifestations of T1DM on gradual loss of pancreatic β cells.

higher than 11·1 mmol/L (200 mg/dL) at random while experiencing manifestations, or a negative oral glucose tolerance examination result. Type 1 diabetes management techniques are still being refined [36]. Tight glucose control has a significant positive impact on individuals with type 1 diabetes. Maintaining strict blood glucose control significantly reduces the risk of both microvascular (such as neuropathy, nephropathy, and retinopathy) and macrovascular (such as myocardial infarction, cerebrovascular accident, and mortality from cardiovascular disease) complications [37]. For the best glycaemic control, multiple-dose insulin regimens that imitate the release of insulin from the body are needed. These regimens should include basal insulin for control during the night and in between meals, as well as bolus doses of rapid-acting insulin analogues to treat hyperglycemia and cover ingested carbohydrate loads [36].

2.2 Importance of diet and nutrition

Type 1 diabetes (T1D) must be managed with a healthy diet, and home-cooked meals can be satisfying and nutrient-dense. Meal documentation in the form of pictures or notes can support dietary consistency. Vegetable incorporation can be more tempting when one participates in activities such as online cookery lessons. The CDC suggests making the same nutritious meals for the whole family rather than depending solely on pricey and frequently disagreeable "diabetic" items. Including plant-based substitutes for meat, such as lentils and beans, provides a wholesome option. Adding vegetables to meals instead of grains or pasta can also improve their nutritious content. Children with type 1 diabetes mellitus (T1DM) frequently lived for years on rigorous carbohydrate restriction prior to the discovery of insulin. The introduction of insulin therapy led to an increase in carbohydrate intake despite a lack of evidence from clinical trials to support its superiority. A low-fat diet that derived up to 60% of its energy from carbohydrates was the norm by the 1980s [38]. The American Diabetes Association (ADA) changed its emphasis from macronutrient objectives to customised dietary strategies. Interest in carbohydrate-modified diets for type 1 diabetes has increased because it has been shown that carbohydrate consumption considerably affects glycaemic variability and postprandial hyperglycemia. Low glycaemic index foods may be able to moderately lower HbA1c by about 0.5%, according to studies. Furthermore, because very low-carb diets (VLCDs) lower postprandial glycemia and require less insulin, they may help T1DM patients achieve remarkable glycaemic control with a lower risk of adverse events [38].

2.3 Physical activity and its effects on glucose metabolism

Frequent exercise enhances weight management, musculoskeletal and cardiometabolic health, and cognitive and psychosocial functioning and is linked to a lower risk of death from diabetes [39]. The Centers for Disease Control and Prevention (CDC) stresses the value of incorporating physical activity into regular activities like using the stairs. Step counts can be increased every day, and progress can be tracked with the use of free tools such as activity trackers. Online exercise videos also offer a range of fitness options appropriate for all skill levels, which makes it simpler for people with T1D to maintain an active lifestyle and enhance their health. Increased insulin delivery following explosive activity, resistance exercise, and/or high-intensity interval training may be useful if hyperglycemia occurs. Nevertheless, continuous glucose monitoring is necessary because the risk of post-exercise hypoglycaemia is increased in the 12 to 24 hours following exercise [39].

2.4 Psychological and emotional aspects

People with T1D frequently experience depression [40]. Individuals with type 1 diabetes (T1D) have much higher rates of psychosocial difficulties than the general population, including depression (2–3 times more likely) and an elevated risk of suicide (3–4 times greater). Up to 40% suffer diabetes-related sadness, which is exacerbated by feelings of pessimism and low self-esteem [41]. Early diagnosis of T1D may cause rebellious behaviour and poor eating habits, which can cause disputes with parents at the dinner table. Such encounters may have an impact on dietary decisions [13]. Treatment for children with T1D who experience moderate depressive episodes is necessary [40]. According to research, adolescents with type 1 diabetes (T1D) have a much greater incidence of depressive symptoms than their peers without the disease. These symptoms have an adverse effect on glycaemic control and diabetes management, in addition to sleep disruptions. Studies addressing these interactions in adolescents with type 1 diabetes are scarce despite the clear correlation between poor sleep, depressed symptoms, and diabetes outcomes (**Figure 3**).

Type 1 diabetes (T1D), once thought to be a childhood ailment, is now more widely diagnosed in adults, with more than half of new cases occurring after the age of 18. Despite this, research and awareness efforts have primarily focused on children, ignoring the psychosocial issues that adults confront, such as stress, identity transformations, and life modifications upon diagnosis [43]. Moreover, psychological comorbidities worsen inadequate glycaemic control, indicating a reciprocal link between sleep problems and diabetes control [44]. Managing stress and ensuring adequate sleep are crucial for individuals with type 1 diabetes (T1D). The U.S. Centers for Disease Control and Prevention (CDC) suggests practices like meditation, yoga, and physical activity, such as walking, to help reduce stress. Social support from friends who understand your situation is also beneficial. For optimal sleep, creating a cool, dark bedroom environment (around 65°F) is recommended. Limiting screen time before bed and engaging in physical activity during the day can improve sleep quality. Establishing a calming bedtime routine, such as taking a shower or reading, further promotes restful sleep, supporting overall diabetes management.

2.5 Complexity of T1D management

The management of Type 1 Diabetes (T1D) is a complex condition because of the interaction of multiple elements, such as biological, psychological, and socioeconomic factors. Continuous self-management is necessary to treat the condition, and it can be particularly difficult in children and adolescents due to their increased risk of having poor glycaemic control [45, 46]. Studies show that the incidence of T1D is rising by 1.9% per year in this group, emphasising the critical need for efficient management techniques [45]. The self-management of type 1 diabetes is greatly impacted by social inequities, which include differences in health literacy, access to medical resources, and support networks [47]. Families are also important in managing diabetes, as disagreements can have a detrimental effect on treatment compliance and general glycaemic control [48]. These factors make focused family interventions necessary to enhance the results of self-management. Patients with type 1 diabetes have dynamic insulin requirements that can vary greatly based on food consumption, stress levels, physical activity, and sickness. Because of this unpredictability, maintaining the best possible glycaemic control necessitates ongoing monitoring and insulin dosage modifications [49, 50]. Moreover, the hazards of hyperglycemia and hypoglycaemia must be

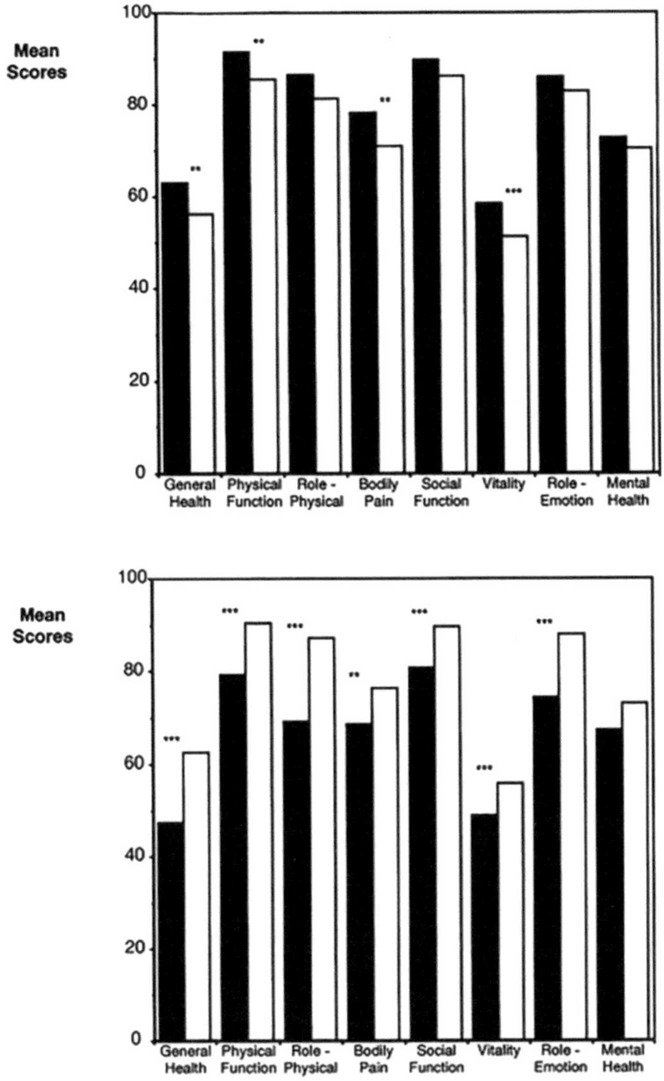

Figure 3.
Two bar graphs show the mean SF-36 scores for various health modalities in persons with Type 1 diabetes. The upper panel splits the data by gender, and the lower panel divides it by household income. Females have lower mental health scores than males. This suggests that female patients with Type 1 diabetes may face increased psychological anguish or emotional issues. Worse household income (<$20,000/year) correlates with worse scores in general health, physical function, role-physical, bodily pain, social function, and mental health compared to higher income groups. This implies that socioeconomic variables could aggravate the health problems associated with Type 1 diabetes. Lower social function scores for both low-income and females indicate that diabetes may have a negative impact on social interactions and relationships. This could be due to issues with body image, fear of judgement, or the need to prioritise diabetes control over social activities. Lower role-emotional scores for low-income people indicate that diabetes may impair their capacity to complete emotional responsibilities, such as being a parent or partner. This could be related to weariness, stress, or the emotional toll of the condition. [Source: Lloyd and Orchard [42]. Physical and psychological well-being in adults with type 1 diabetes.]

carefully balanced in T1DM therapy. While strict glycaemic management can lower the chance of microvascular (such as retinopathy and nephropathy) and macrovascular problems in the long run, it can also raise the risk of hypoglycaemia episodes [50, 51]. Effective T1DM management requires a comprehensive strategy that includes dietary, psychological, and physical support. In order to address the distinct obstacles that each patient experiences, healthcare practitioners need to take these factors into account while creating individualised treatment regimens [52].

2.6 Emphasis on the critical role of insulin therapy

Since Type 1 Diabetes Mellitus (T1DM) is characterised by the autoimmune death of insulin-producing pancreatic beta cells, which leads to insulin insufficiency, insulin therapy is a crucial part of managing the condition. Patients can control their blood glucose levels and avoid the condition's acute and long-term consequences by administering insulin correctly. People who do not take enough insulin run the danger of developing severe hyperglycemia, which can result in diabetic ketoacidosis and possibly be fatal [53]. The majority of T1DM patients use continuous subcutaneous insulin infusion (CSII) systems or multiple daily injections (MDI) of both basal and bolus insulin. While prandial insulins control blood glucose rises during meals, basal insulins, like their long-acting counterparts, maintain glucose levels in between meals. This method closely resembles the physiological secretion of insulin, which is essential for efficient glycaemic management [53]. Optimised glycaemic objectives, usually a HbA1c level of less than 7%, require patient education on carb counting and individualised treatment programmes that are guided by regular blood glucose monitoring. Additionally, continuous glucose monitoring (CGM) devices have become essential tools that improve treatment adherence and overall quality of life by boosting the capacity to identify and manage hypoglycaemia [53].

3. Innovations in diabetes management

Patient outcomes have improved dramatically as a result of recent developments in the therapy of Type 1 Diabetes (T1D). Important developments include insulin pump therapy, especially hybrid closed-loop systems that improve glycaemic control and offer real-time data, and continuous glucose monitoring (CGM) devices. Furthermore, postprandial glucose regulation has been enhanced by ultrarapid-acting insulins and supplementary treatments such as SGLT2 inhibitors and GLP-1 receptor agonists. Better self-management has been encouraged by the expansion of information and assistance available through digital health platforms and telemedicine. When taken as a whole, these developments are revolutionising the way T1D is managed, lessening its impact, and enhancing the lives of those who have the illness [54].

3.1 Technological developments transforming treatment paradigms

The treatment paradigms for Type 1 Diabetes (T1D) are being profoundly altered by technological breakthroughs, which improve patient outcomes and self-management. Innovations such as continuous glucose monitoring and insulin delivery systems are changing the way people with type 1 diabetes live. Although exogenous insulin has long been the mainstay of T1D care, the development of insulin pumps that are controlled by glucose sensors has completely changed the way insulin is administered [55, 56]. By automating insulin delivery in response to real-time glucose measurements, these pumps lessen the need for continuous monitoring and enhance glycaemic management [57]. The introduction of continuous glucose monitoring (CGM) systems, which offer continuous insights into blood glucose levels, is a result of technological improvements in diabetes management [58]. With the help of this technology, blood glucose can be actively managed, allowing users to more precisely modify insulin dosages and prevent problems. Pancreatic islet transplantation is one example of an innovation that has changed the lives of those with severe T1D who are at risk of hypoglycaemia [59, 60]. These therapies, which aim to address immunological issues and enhance long-term outcomes, are at the forefront of diabetes care; however, they are currently undergoing research and development. The treatment and results for kids and teenagers with type 1 diabetes have significantly improved over the last few decades, primarily because of technological advancements [61]. These developments improve patients' quality of life and dramatically lower their likelihood of developing serious diabetes-related complications. The field of T1D treatment is changing, and this represents an evolution towards more individualised and efficient care [62]. The use of cutting-edge technologies not only simplifies the management of diabetes but also gives individuals greater control over their health.

3.2 Advances in insulin delivery systems

If accessible, insulin can be injected using an insulin pen; otherwise, an insulin pump is the preferred method for most people [36]. The integration of many devices, such as insulin pumps and connected insulin pens, has been observed in recent advancements in insulin delivery. Continuous glucose monitoring and insulin delivery are made possible by these sophisticated systems, enabling real-time data processing and insulin titration according to each patient's unique metabolic requirements [63]. With the use of continuous glucose monitoring (CGM) technology, patients can monitor their blood sugar levels continuously throughout the day without having to often puncture their skin [64]. A revolutionary change in the treatment of diabetes is represented by the automated insulin delivery devices. By employing predictive algorithms to modify insulin delivery in response to real-time glucose measurements, these devices resemble "artificial pancreas" functions [65]. Significant gains in the amount of time spent within target glucose ranges have been shown by AID systems, which improve overall glycaemic management and lessen the need for manual insulin dose adjustments [66, 67]. Another noteworthy development is the availability of insulin analogues with ultra-rapid action. When these formulations are incorporated into both closed- and open-loop delivery systems, postprandial hyperglycemia can be better controlled. Studies conducted in clinical settings have demonstrated that significant improvements in glycaemic outcomes can be obtained by modifying medication parameters to account for these quicker insulin analogues, hence raising the bar for patient care [68].

4. Building daily resilience

4.1 Establishing a supportive network of family, friends, and healthcare providers

For people with Type 1 Diabetes (T1D) to develop everyday resilience, they must create a network of family, friends, and healthcare providers. These networks improve coping strategies and general well-being by offering emotional, practical, and informative assistance. Friends and family can foster a supportive atmosphere that promotes candid discussions about managing diabetes, which lessens feelings of loneliness and anxiety [69, 70]. Social networks can also strengthen a feeling of belonging, which is important for mental well-being [70]. Healthcare providers are essential to this supportive system because they give specialised medical care and professional guidance to individuals with T1D. Consultations on a regular basis facilitate efficient diabetes treatment and give access to tools that improve self-management abilities [71]. Furthermore, a cooperative approach between patients and healthcare providers can greatly enhance the quality of patient outcomes [72]. In conclusion, building robust support systems improves long-term resilience and health outcomes in addition to improving the day-to-day management of Type 1 Diabetes. Over time, the bonds formed through supportive interactions can improve both psychological and physical health by acting as a buffer against stressors related to diabetes [73, 74].

5. Conclusion

Managing Type 1 diabetes (T1D) entails many difficulties, ranging from insulin therapy and blood glucose regulation to lifestyle, psychological, and emotional aspects. Diabetes care has been completely transformed by technological advancements in insulin pumps, continuous glucose monitoring (CGM) devices, hybrid closed-loop systems, and ultrarapid-acting insulins. The complexity of the condition remains despite these advancements, requiring ongoing monitoring and modifications to insulin levels, food, and exercise. The management of T1D patients is further complicated by social, psychological, and economic variables. These patients frequently experience increased rates of despair, stress, and sleep difficulties. In order to avoid complications such as diabetic ketoacidosis, early identification is essential, and long-term treatment must take mental and physical health into account. Effective T1D management requires comprehensive and individualised treatment strategies that include nutritional, medical, psychological, and physical support. Comprehending the complex characteristics of type 1 diabetes, ranging from hereditary and environmental origins to its influence on everyday living, highlights the necessity of ongoing study and innovation in enhancing patient outcomes.

Acknowledgements

I want to acknowledge everyone who contributed to this chapter from the bottom of my heart. A special thank you to my co-workers for their insightful advice and encouragement during the composition process. I am also profoundly grateful for my family's consistent support and understanding. Ultimately, I express my gratitude to the readers whose engagement and curiosity have motivated our work. This chapter would not have been possible without everyone's assistance and combined efforts. We appreciate your support in making this idea a reality and the conviction you hold in it.

Abbreviations

T1DM	type 1 diabetes
CGM	continuous glucose monitoring
%	percentage
WHO	world health organisation
AAb	autoantibodies

GAD	glutamic acid decarboxylase
CSII	continuous subcutaneous insulin infusion
ATP	adenosine triphosphate
DKA	diabetic ketoacidosis
CDCP	centres for disease control and prevention
ADA	American diabetes association
HbA1c	glycated haemoglobin
VLCDs	very low-carb diets
SGLT2	sodium-glucose cotransporter-2
GLP-1	glucagon-like peptide-1
β	beta
MDI	multiple daily injections

Author details

Yashika Saini[1], Mohseen[2*] and Rajesh Kumar Sharma[2]

1 School of Life and Basic Science, Jaipur National University, Jaipur, Rajasthan, India

2 Department of Pharmacology, Nims Institute of Pharmacy, Nims University, Jaipur, Rajasthan, India

*Address all correspondence to: mohseenalimomeen@gmail.com

References

[1] Pratley RE, Kanapka LG, Rickels MR, Ahmann A, Aleppo G, Beck R, et al. Effect of continuous glucose monitoring on hypoglycemia in older adults with type 1 diabetes: A randomized clinical trial. JAMA. 2020;**323**(23):2397-2406

[2] James EA, Joglekar AV, Linnemann AK, Russ HA, Kent SC. The beta cell-immune cell interface in type 1 diabetes (T1D). Molecular Metabolism. 2023:101809

[3] Mazzilli R, Imbrogno N, Elia J, Delfino M, Bitterman O, Napoli A, et al. Sexual dysfunction in diabetic women: Prevalence and differences in type 1 and type 2 diabetes mellitus. Diabetes, Metabolic Syndrome and Obesity: Targets and Therapy. 2015;**11**:97-101

[4] Nieto T, Castillo B, Nieto J, Redondo MJ. Demographic and diagnostic markers in new onset pediatric type 1 and type 2 diabetes: Differences and overlaps. Annals of Pediatric Endocrinology & Metabolism. 2022;**27**(2):121

[5] Wallace AS, Chang AR, Shin JI, Reider J, Echouffo-Tcheugui JB, Grams ME, et al. Obesity and chronic kidney disease in US adults with type 1 and type 2 diabetes mellitus. The Journal of Clinical Endocrinology & Metabolism. 2022;**107**(5):1247-1256

[6] Hartmann B, Tittel SR, Femerling M, Pfeifer M, Meyhöfer S, Lange K, et al. COVID-19 lockdown periods in 2020: Good maintenance of metabolic control in adults with type 1 and type 2 diabetes. Experimental and Clinical Endocrinology & Diabetes: Official Journal, German Society of Endocrinology [and] German Diabetes Association. 2022;**130**:621-626

[7] Petrova NL, Foster AV, Edmonds ME. Calcaneal bone mineral density in patients with Charcot neuropathic osteoarthropathy: Differences between type 1 and type 2 diabetes. Diabetic Medicine. 2005;**22**:756-761

[8] Idris I, Gordon J, Tilling C, Vora JP. A cost comparison of long-acting insulin analogs vs NPH insulin-based treatment in patients with type 2 diabetes using routinely collected primary care data from the UK. Journal of Medical Economics. 2015;**18**:273-282

[9] Zaccardi F, Webb DR, Yates T, Davies MJ. Pathophysiology of type 1 and type 2 diabetes mellitus: A 90-year perspective. Postgraduate Medical Journal. 2016;**92**(1084):63-69

[10] de Souza ABC, Correa-Giannella MLC, Gomes MB, Negrato CA, Nery M. Epidemiology and risk factors of hypoglycemia in subjects with type 1 diabetes in Brazil: A cross-sectional, multicenter study. Archives of Endocrinology and Metabolism. 2022;**66**(6):784-791

[11] American Diabetes Association. Hypoglycemia (low blood sugar). Diabetes Care. 2023;**46**(Suppl. 1):S45-S50

[12] Zajec A, Trebušak Podkrajšek K, Tesovnik T, Šket R, Čugalj Kern B, Jenko Bizjan B, et al. Pathogenesis of type 1 diabetes: Established facts and new insights. Genes. 2022;**13**(4):706

[13] Goldberg T, Brener A, Levy S, Interator H, Laurian I, Dorfman A, et al. Association between age at type 1 diabetes diagnosis and metabolic outcome at young adulthood: A real-life observational study. Diabetes/Metabolism Research and Reviews. 2021;**37**(1):e3356

[14] Kaul K, Apostolopoulou M, Roden M. Insulin resistance in type 1 diabetes mellitus. Metabolism. 2015;**64**(12):1629-1639

[15] American Diabetes Association. Diagnosis and classification of diabetes mellitus. Diabetes Care. 2014;**37** (Suppl. 1):S81-S90

[16] Gale EAM. The discovery of type 1 diabetes. Diabetologia. 2013;**56**(10):2200-2213

[17] Rosenbloom AL. Hyperglycemic emergencies in children with diabetes mellitus. Pediatric Clinics of North America. 2010;**52**(6):1639-1653

[18] Boden G. Role of fatty acids in the pathogenesis of insulin resistance and NIDDM. Diabetes. 1997;**46**(1):3-10

[19] Muller LM, Gorter KJ, Hak E, Goudzwaard WL, Schellevis FG, Hoepelman AIM, et al. Increased risk of common infections in patients with type 1 and type 2 diabetes mellitus. Clinical Infectious Diseases. 2017;**41**(3):281-288

[20] Chiang JL, Kirkman MS, Laffel LMB, Peters AL. Type 1 diabetes through the life span: A position statement of the American Diabetes Association. Diabetes Care. 2014;**37**(7):2034-2054

[21] Mazzone T, Chait A, Plutzky J. Cardiovascular disease risk in type 2 diabetes mellitus: Insights from mechanistic studies. The Lancet. 2008;**371**(9626):1800-1809

[22] Nakhoul NF, Abdul-Ghani M. Pathogenesis of hypertension in diabetes: A comprehensive physiology review. Journal of Diabetes and its Complications. 2018;**32**(6):488-497

[23] Callaghan BC, Cheng HT, Stables CL, Smith AL, Feldman EL. Diabetic neuropathy: Clinical manifestations and current treatments. The Lancet Neurology. 2012;**11**(6):521-534

[24] Nitzan O, Elias M, Chazan B, Saliba W. Urinary tract infections in patients with type 2 diabetes mellitus: Review of prevalence, diagnosis, and management. Diabetes, Metabolic Syndrome and Obesity: Targets and Therapy. 2015;**8**:129-136

[25] Saran R, Li Y, Robinson B, Ayanian J, Balkrishnan R, Bragg-Gresham J, et al. US renal data system 2014 annual data report: Epidemiology of kidney disease in the United States. American Journal of Kidney Diseases. 2015;**66**(1):305

[26] Li X, Zarbin MA, Bhagat N. Cataract surgery in patients with diabetes mellitus. The American Journal of Ophthalmology. 2014;**157**(5):1041-1049

[27] Yau JWY, Rogers SL, Kawasaki R, Lamoureux EL, Kowalski JW, Bek T, et al. Global prevalence and major risk factors of diabetic retinopathy. Diabetes Care. 2012;**35**(3):556-564

[28] Horowitz M, Edelbroek MA, Fraser R, Maddox A. Disordered gastric motor function in diabetes mellitus. Diabetologia. 2012;**37**(6):543-551

[29] Parkman HP, Yates KP, Hasler WL, Nguyan L, Pasricha PJ, Snape WJ, et al. Similarities and differences between diabetic and idiopathic gastroparesis. Clinical Gastroenterology and Hepatology. 2010;**9**(12):1056-1064

[30] Vestergaard P. Discrepancies in bone mineral density and fracture risk in patients with type 1 and type 2 diabetes: A meta-analysis. Osteoporosis International. 2007;**18**(4):427-444

[31] Starup-Linde J, Eriksen SA, Lykkeboe S, Handberg A, Vestergaard P,

Gregersen S. Biochemical markers of bone turnover in diabetes patients—A meta-analysis, and a methodological study on the effects of glucose on bone markers. Osteoporosis International. 2016;**27**(4):1697-1706

[32] Atkinson MA. The pathogenesis and natural history of type 1 diabetes. Cold Spring Harbor Perspectives in Medicine. 2012;**2**(11):a007641

[33] Vaglio A, Grayson PC, Hoffman GS. Recent advances in the research and management of relapsing polychondritis and vasculitis. Current Opinion in Rheumatology. 2017;**29**(1):1-9

[34] Hackett G. The burden and extent of comorbid erectile dysfunction in type 2 diabetes. The Journal of Sexual Medicine. 2015;**12**(4):829-846

[35] Kim C, Liske JC, Fontaine P, Wolfe K. Type 1 diabetes in pregnancy. Current Obstetrics and Gynecology Reports. 2016;**5**(1):29-38

[36] DiMeglio LA, Evans-Molina C, Oram RA. Type 1 diabetes. The Lancet. 2018;**391**(10138):2449-2462

[37] Smith A, Harris C. Type 1 diabetes: management strategies. American Family Physician. 2018;**98**(3):154-162

[38] Lennerz BS, Barton A, Bernstein RK, Dikeman RD, Diulus C, Hallberg S, et al. Management of type 1 diabetes with a very low–carbohydrate diet. Pediatrics. 2018;**141**(6):e20173349

[39] Riddell MC, Peters AL. Exercise in adults with type 1 diabetes mellitus. Nature Reviews Endocrinology. 2023;**19**(2):98-111

[40] Herman H, Ardani IGAI, Aryani LNA, Windiani IGAT, Adnyana IGNS, Setiawati Y. Signs and symptoms of depression in children and adolescents with type 1 diabetes mellitus: A case report. International Journal of Health and Medical Sciences. 2022;**5**(1):150-153

[41] Kelly RC, Holt RI, Desborough L, Majidi S, Town M, Naranjo D, et al. The psychosocial burdens of living with diabetes. Diabetic Medicine. 2024;**41**(3):e15219

[42] Lloyd CE, Orchard TJ. Physical and psychological well-being in adults with type 1 diabetes. Diabetes Research and Clinical Practice. 1999;**44**(1):9-19

[43] Due-Christensen M, Bruun LD, Joensen LE, Norgaard O, Andersen TH. Psychosocial aspects and perspectives of adult-onset type 1 diabetes: A systematic scoping review. Diabetic Medicine. 2023;**40**(5):e15073

[44] Hamburger ER, Goethals ER, Choudhary A, Jaser SS. Sleep and depressive symptoms in adolescents with type 1 diabetes not meeting glycemic targets. Diabetes Research and Clinical Practice. 2020;**169**:108442

[45] Granados A, Carrillo Iregui A. Type 1 diabetes Management in the Hospital Setting. Pediatrics in Review. 2024;**45**(4):201-209

[46] Wilson V. Managing type 1 diabetes in children and young people: Challenges and solutions. Nursing Children and Young People. 2023;**35**:35-42. DOI: 10.7748/ncyp.2023.e1465. Advance online publication

[47] Wagner S, Olesen K. Social inequalities in the self-management of type 1 diabetes: A serial multiple mediation analysis. Scandinavian Journal of Public Health. 2021;**51**:250-256

[48] Vaid E, Lansing AH, Stanger C. Problems with self-regulation, family

conflict, and glycemic control in adolescents experiencing challenges with managing type 1 diabetes. Journal of Pediatric Psychology. 2018;**43**(5):525-533

[49] Colberg SR. Practical Management of Type 1 diabetes during exercise. Journal of Physical Education, Recreation & Dance. 2000;**71**(2):24-27

[50] Zekarias KL, Seaquist ER. Prevalence of Hypoglycemia in Patients with Type 1 Diabetes and Advanced Type 2 Diabetes. SMGroup; 2017

[51] Sudan SS, Batra B. Available treatments for type 2 diabetes: A REVIEW. International Journal of Engineering Applied Sciences and Technology. 2020;**5**:572-577

[52] Oliveira GY, Lima FD, Souza NP, Sabino LM, Freitas CH, Veras VS. Nursing care to people with type 1 diabetes in intensive care: Integrative review. Journal of Nursing Ufpe Online. 2016;**10**:3438-3445

[53] Janež A, Guja C, Mitrakou A, Lalic N, Tankova T, Czupryniak L, et al. Insulin therapy in adults with type 1 diabetes mellitus: A narrative review. Diabetes Therapy. 2020;**11**:387-409

[54] Bahal M, Pande V, Dua J, Mane S. Advances in type 1 diabetes mellitus management in children. Cureus. 2024;**16**(8):e67377

[55] Kobayati A, Haidar A, Tsoukas MA. Glucagon-like peptide-1 receptor agonists as adjunctive treatment for type 1 diabetes: Renewed opportunities through tailored approaches? Diabetes, Obesity & Metabolism. 2022;**24**(5):769-787

[56] de Valk HW. Insulinepomp aangestuurd door een glucosesensor [Insulin pump regulated by a glucose sensor; one step closer to closing the loop for type 1 diabetes patients]. Nederlands Tijdschrift voor Geneeskunde. 2019;**163**:D3713

[57] Valk HW. Insulin pump regulated by a glucose sensor; one step closer to closing the loop for type 1 diabetes patients. Nederlands Tijdschrift voor Geneeskunde. 2019;**163**:D3713

[58] Ferenci T, Körner A, Kovács L. Correlation investigations between HbAlc and blood glucose indicators on type 1 diabetic Hungarian children. In: 2013 IEEE 8th International Symposium on Applied Computational Intelligence and Informatics (SACI). Timisoara, Romania; 2013. pp. 443-447

[59] Ho BX, Teo AKK, Ng NHJ. Innovations in bio-engineering and cell-based approaches to address immunological challenges in islet transplantation. Frontiers in Immunology. 2024;**15**:1375177

[60] Bolla AM, Montefusco L, Pastore I, Lunati ME, Ben Nasr M, Fiorina P. Benefits and hurdles of pancreatic β-cell replacement. Stem Cells Translational Medicine. 2022;**11**:1029-1039

[61] Fairchild JM. Changes in management and outcomes for children and adolescents with type 1 diabetes over the last 50 years. Journal of Paediatrics and Child Health. 2015;**51**:122-125

[62] Gunatilake SSC. Technological innovations in type 1 diabetes mellitus management: A narrative review. Sri Lanka Journal of Diabetes Endocrinology and Metabolism. 2024;**15**:17-24

[63] Yoo JH, Kim JH. Advances in continuous glucose monitoring and integrated devices for management of diabetes with insulin-based therapy: Improvement in glycemic control. Diabetes & Metabolism Journal. 2023;**47**(1):27-41

[64] Nwokolo M, Hovorka R. The artificial pancreas and type 1 diabetes. The Journal of Clinical Endocrinology and Metabolism. 2023;**108**:1614-1623

[65] Nefs G. The psychological implications of automated insulin delivery Systems in Type 1 diabetes care. Frontiers in Clinical Diabetes and Healthcare. 2022;**3**:1-6

[66] Perkins BA, Sherr JL, Mathieu C. Type 1 diabetes glycemic management: Insulin therapy, glucose monitoring, and automation. Science. 2021;**373**:522-527

[67] Lee TTM, Collett C, Bergford S, Hartnell S, Scott E, Lindsay RS, et al. Automated closed-loop insulin delivery for the management of type 1 diabetes during pregnancy: The AiDAPT RCT. Efficacy and Mechanism Evaluation. 2024;**11**:1-80

[68] Diaz J, Colmegna P, Breton MD. Maximizing glycemic benefits of using faster insulin formulations in type 1 diabetes: In-silico analysis under open- and closed-loop conditions. Diabetes Technology & Therapeutics. 2023;**25**:219-230

[69] Hill K, Ward P, Gleadle J. “I kind of gave up on it after a while, became too hard, closed my eyes, didn't want to know about it”—Adults with type 1 diabetes mellitus describe defeat in the context of low social support. Health Expectations. 2019;**22**(2):254-261

[70] Shah LL, Ersig AL, Paik A. Social network factors and anxiety among adolescents with type 1 diabetes and their parents. Journal of Family Nursing. 2019;**25**(3):395-418

[71] Araujo ACMC, Mesquita IM, Silva AP, Dias AMCB, Ribeiro FA, Tom JM, et al. Relationship between resilience, self-care and metabolic control in patients with type 1 diabetes mellitus. Journal Archives of Health. 2024;**5**(2):e1640-e1640

[72] Scott SR, O’Donnell M, Manczak EM, Fladeboe K, Ellisor B, Rosenberg AR, et al. Resilience and diabetes distress at 3 months following diagnosis predict A1C trajectories in youth with type 1 diabetes: An argument for early intervention. Journal of Pediatric Psychology. 2022;**47**(10):1125-1134

[73] Koegelenberg G. Resilience Characteristics of Families with a Child with Type 1 Diabetes. Stellenbosch: Stellenbosch University; 2013

[74] Whitaker RC, Dearth-Wesley T, Herman AN, Nagel KE, Smith HG, Weil HF. Association of childhood family connection with flourishing in young adulthood among those with type 1 diabetes. JAMA Network Open. 2020;**3**(3):e200427-e200427

Chapter 6

Dietary Advanced Glycation End-Products (AGES) Induced Complications in Type 1 Diabetes Mellitus

Sanchari Bhattacharyya and Sagar Acharya

Abstract

The buildup of advanced glycation end-products (AGEs) in the diet is a significant factor that contributes to the worsening of problems linked with type 1 diabetes mellitus (T1D). This chapter explores the role of advanced glycation end-products (AGEs) in type 1 diabetes mellitus (T1D) complications. AGEs are produced during food cooking and processing, leading to the accumulation of AGEs in the body. These AGEs exacerbate oxidative stress and inflammation by interacting with the receptor for AGEs (RAGE), activating pro-inflammatory and pro-fibrotic signalling pathways. AGEs contribute to microvascular and macrovascular issues in T1D, affecting renal, cardiovascular, and retinal disorders. They cause structural and functional changes in tissues, leading to glomerular damage, endothelial dysfunction, and brain injury. Persistent oxidative stress and inflammation increase insulin resistance and compromise glycemic control. The chapter emphasises the importance of dietary measures to reduce AGE consumption, the negative effects on health, and therapeutic approaches targeting AGE synthesis and RAGE signalling to ameliorate type 1 diabetes mellitus-associated complications.

Keywords: advanced glycation end-products (AGEs), dietary AGEs, type 1 diabetes mellitus, oxidative stress, inflammation, RAGE, renal complications, cardiovascular complications, retinal complications, diabetic complications, dietary strategies, therapeutic interventions

1. Introduction

Type 1 diabetes mellitus (T1D) is an autoimmune disease in which the immune system attacks the beta cells in the pancreas that make insulin. This causes the body to not make enough insulin. It comes on quickly and does not have any antibodies tied to diabetes. The onset of T1D has many reasons, some of which are genetic, like certain HLA haplotypes and MHC class I genes, and some of which are environmental. Genetic susceptibility is different between Asian and Caucasian groups, as shown by studies that show different people have different clinical and autoimmunity traits [1]. Most cases are caused by an autoimmune process that destroys beta cells (type 1a), but some cases are caused by beta cells failing or being destroyed for no apparent reason. T1D makes up 5–10% of all cases of diabetes in the world. One hypothesis is that people get T1D because of their genes, and the other is that their genes are influenced by their surroundings [2].

Advanced glycation end products, or AGEs, are a group of different chemicals that are made when reducing sugars combine with proteins, lipids, or nucleic acids without the help of enzymes. AGEs attach to one or more of their many receptors (RAGE) found on different types of cells. This sets off a chain of biological reactions that are detrimental to the health of the individual [3]. According to research, when AGE and its receptor (RAGE) connect, reactive oxygen species (ROS) are created, which in turn cause oxidative stress. High blood sugar makes AGE development worse because AGE is mostly made when glucose in the blood spontaneously oxidises [4]. Here, we will dive into the details of AGEs, how they are formed, how they interact with their receptors on the surface of different cells, and the signalling pathways activated by them. We will also explore more about the different complications caused by dietary AGEs in individuals already suffering from T1D and the steps that can be taken to reduce the effects of these dietary AGEs in such scenarios. Our objective is to investigate how such AGEs impact cellular processes and contribute to the course of diseases. Through this examination, we want to uncover possible treatment approaches and dietary changes that might help reduce these harmful consequences. Gaining insight into the influence of dietary AGEs on the management of T1D is essential for creating all-encompassing care strategies that enhance long-term health results for individuals suffering from this disease.

2. Advanced glycation end-products (AGEs)

2.1 AGEs and their formation

AGEs are chemicals formed through non-enzymatic interactions between reducing sugars and lipids, proteins, or nucleic acids. They are formed through non-enzymatic condensation, a process without a biological catalyst. This reaction involves carbonyl groups of reducing sugars and free amine groups of nucleic acids, lipids, or proteins. AGEs can also be created through the traditional Maillard process, also known as the browning reaction. Other processes, such as oxidation of sugars, lipids, and amino acids, also contribute to AGE formation.

2.2 Maillard reaction

The Maillard reaction is a crucial biological process that causes enzymatic browning and enhances the flavour of prepared meals. Discovered by French scientist Louis-Camille Maillard in the early twentieth century, it is important in culinary and scientific contexts due to its impact on food flavour, colour, nutrition, and health. Hodge simplified the reaction into three major stages: a reversible condensation reaction, dehydration and fragmentation, and condensation reactions. The first stage involves a reducing sugar interacting with an amino acid, resulting in an unstable Schiff's base. The second stage involves dehydration and fragmentation, forming reactive intermediate compounds like dicarbonyl compounds. The final stages lead to melanoidins, brown, nitrogenous polymers, and co-polymers, responsible for food browning [5]. These reactive intermediates, known as AGEs, are crucial for producing

DOI: http://dx.doi.org/10.5772/intechopen.1007016

complex tastes in cooked food and can cause oxidative stress, which can have detrimental health effects. The detailed Maillard reaction is shown in **Figure 1**.

2.3 Endogenous AGEs

Endogenous AGEs are substances produced in the body through chemical interactions between reducing sugars and proteins, lipids, or nucleic acids without enzymes. They play a role in ageing and chronic diseases like diabetes, cardiovascular disease, and neurological illnesses. The Maillard reaction, a component of regular metabolic processes, contributes to cellular function and signalling. It is typically regulated and maintained at minimal levels during normal physiological circumstances. If left unchecked, AGEs build up in body tissues and organs gradually, particularly in cases of high blood sugar levels, such as those seen in diabetes [6].

2.4 Exogenous AGEs

Exogenous AGEs, produced outside the body through cooking and processing, are consumed through food and contribute to the body's accumulation. These AGEs are produced by the Maillard reaction and are found in protein and fat-rich meals like meat, cheese, and processed foods. Understanding dietary AGEs is crucial as they can worsen health issues like diabetes. Accumulating AGEs alters protein structure and function, creating cross-links, and can increase tissue rigidity and decrease functionality, particularly for long-lived proteins like collagen [7].

2.5 Regulation of AGEs in the body

AGEs, both endogenous and exogenous, are produced in the body through various mechanisms. The glyoxalase system removes reactive dicarbonyl compounds, like methylglyoxal, from the body through the conversion of glyoxalase I and II into

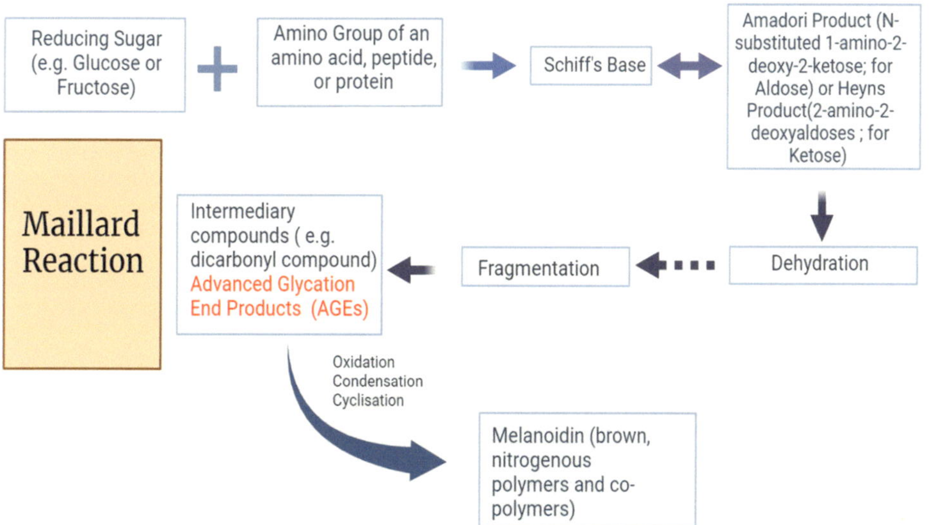

Figure 1.
Maillard reaction that results in the formation of advanced glycation end products (AGEs).

D-lactate [8–10]. Amadoriase enzymes convert early glycation products into less reactive molecules, preventing their conversion into more stable AGEs. AGE receptors, such as AGE-R1, AGE-R2, and AGE-R3, neutralise AGEs. Macrophages, possessing scavenger receptor class A and CD36, internalise AGEs into macrophages and destroy them inside lysosomes [11]. AGEs are then eliminated from circulation through endocytosis in the liver and excreted through the kidneys. These molecules cause oxidative stress, and antioxidants like glutathione, superoxide dismutase, and catalase can mitigate this. High intake of vitamins C and E, polyphenols, and flavonoids can also help reduce oxidative stress and inhibit AGE formation [12, 13].

3. Receptors for advanced glycation end products

AGEs interact with particular receptors on the surfaces of cells, controlling their functions and generating anti-glycation effects. There exist two distinct types of receptors: the receptor for advanced glycation end products (RAGE) and the receptor specific to advanced glycation end products (AGER1) [14, 15]. RAGE, an immunoglobulin superfamily member, initiates intracellular signalling pathways that result in inflammation, oxidative damage, and cellular dysfunction. AGER1 functions as a receptor that counteracts glycation by binding to advanced glycation end products (AGEs) and promoting their uptake and degradation. It has been recognised as a safeguarding controller against liver fibrosis in animal models of NASH and type 2 diabetes mellitus. AGE receptors serve to safeguard vital tissues and organs from harm resulting from AGE-induced glycation [16–21]. Gaining a comprehensive understanding of the intricate interplay between these receptors and AGEs is of utmost importance in order to devise effective treatment strategies for tackling AGE-related illnesses, especially in the context of type T1D.

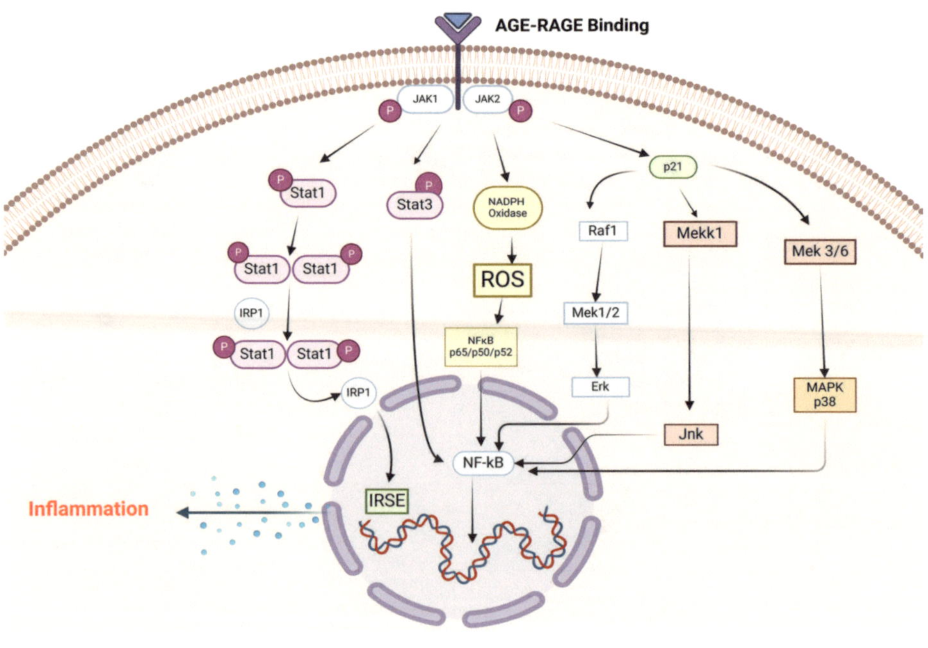

Figure 2.
Signalling pathways activated after AGE-RAGE interaction.

3.1 AGE-RAGE interaction

Many physiological and pathological processes, such as chronic inflammation, oxidative stress, vascular issues, neurodegeneration, and diabetes, can be impacted by the protein RAGE, which is expressed in many cell types. The interaction between AGEs and RAGE triggers a complex network of signalling pathways, including NF-κB, MAPK, JAK/STAT, PI3K/Akt, Rho GTPases, reactive oxygen species (ROS) generation, and transforming growth factor beta (TGF-β) (**Figure 2**). These pathways have a role in the abnormal physiological processes of diabetes and its effects. The binding of AGEs to receptors initiates physiological responses, such as inflammation and the production of free radicals [10, 22–24]. AGEs bind to RAGE, which can then bind to other ligands such as S100A12, S100b, and HMGB1. This binding activates internal signalling pathways and leads to inflammation [22, 25]. This interaction plays a pivotal role in the development of diseases such as diabetes, resulting in persistent inflammation, oxidative stress, decreased blood vessel function, diminished insulin responsiveness, programmed cell death, and excessive creation of fibrous tissue.

4. Type 1 diabetes mellitus and dietary AGEs

T1D accounts for 5–10% of the total number of diabetes cases worldwide. This is a chronic autoimmune illness that causes gradual destruction to the β-cells in the islets of Langerhans in the pancreas. This damage leads to a significant decrease in insulin production, which in turn causes dangerously high levels of glucose in the blood, posing a threat to life. Patients afflicted with this condition typically exhibit typical symptoms like excessive urine (polyuria), exhaustion, and loss of weight. In addition, they have islet-specific antibodies against self-antigens, indicating the presence of pancreatic autoimmunity. Heightened intake of heavily processed foods is a significant environmental factor that can impact the likelihood of developing T1D. Food processing enhances economically advantageous characteristics such as extended shelf-life, enhanced flavour, and improved digestibility, employing techniques such as dry heat baking. However, the presence of increased levels of sugar, fat, refined carbohydrates, and lower levels of whole grains in highly processed diets enhances the development of AGEs. Carboxymethyl lysine (CML) and methyl-glyoxal-derived hydroimidazolones (MG-H1) are the most prevalent and extensively researched ligands of AGEs in living organisms. These ligands have been identified to specifically interact with AGE receptors, including the receptor for advanced glycation end products (RAGE). Research has revealed that dietary items with brief heating durations, low levels of protein and carbs, and high-water content, such as fruits and vegetables, contain the least amount of AGEs. AGEs included in food can be absorbed through the gastrointestinal system, adding to the body's pool of AGEs. According to research conducted on both humans and animals, it is estimated that around 10% of the total AGEs consumed are absorbed into the bloodstream. Out of these, two-thirds are retained in the body for a period exceeding 3 days. Research conducted on mice has shown that consuming dietary AGEs can increase the levels of AGEs in both the bloodstream and tissues.

4.1 Dietary AGEs and their sources

Dietary AGEs are often formed when the Maillard reaction takes place during the cooking process of food at high temperatures or the preparation of processed food.

Cooking practices like grilling raw food directly at high temperatures cause increased content of AGE in food. The browning of grilled food materials is Maillard reaction, which gives the final product as AGE. Similarly, deep frying or pan-frying food, roasting or baking at high temperatures, or microwaving for long periods, can cause accumulation of dietary AGEs, as all these processes lead to Maillard reaction. Below is a list of sources of common dietary AGEs:

i. Beef, chicken, pig, and fish, particularly when prepared using high-temperature cooking methods like grilling, roasting, and frying, contain a significant amount of AGEs.

ii. Processed meats such as sausages, hot dogs, bacon, and other similar products generally have high levels of AGEs as a result of the curing, smoking, and frying methods used in their production.

iii. Hard cheeses such as Parmesan and Cheddar contain a greater amount of AGEs in comparison to softer cheeses. Butter and cream, being dairy fats, contain AGEs, particularly when utilised in the process of cooking or baking.

iv. Processed foods like French fries, potato chips, and commercially baked goods like cookies, cakes, and pastries are prepared using high temperatures while baking and frying are high in AGEs.

v. Fast foods like burgers, pizzas, etc. are prepared by high-temperature grilling and baking, especially topped with processed meat like pepperoni and dairy product cheese is doubly high in AGE content.

vi. Food products high in sugar content like candies, that are caramelised, processed syrup, sweetened sauces, etc. are also high in AGEs, firstly because of the high temperatures used to process these items and second, due to the presence of high quantities of sugar in them.

4.2 Metabolism and absorption of dietary AGEs

Gaining insight into the metabolic process of diet-derived AGEs is crucial for maintaining optimal health. The typical daily consumption of AGEs in adults is around 16,000 AGE kU. Consuming heat-treated meals, high-sugar foods, and highly processed foods like full-fat cheese and meat substantially raises the consumption of AGEs, surpassing 20,000 kU/day [26]. Studies indicate that AGEs can build up and attach to various tissues throughout the body within a 72-hour timeframe. The liver and kidneys are the primary organs where AGEs tend to collect [27, 28]. The process of eliminating AGEs through the kidneys is crucial. AGEs present in food can be absorbed by the human body through the gastrointestinal digestion and absorption process. The absorption rate of AGEs can range from 10% to 30%. It is estimated that around 30% of the total absorbed AGEs are excreted through the kidneys in healthy individuals. However, this percentage decreases to as low as 5% in patients with kidney disease. These findings are based on specific studies that quantified the pure content of AGEs in food [29]. These findings indicate that AGEs in food do not exist in isolation, but rather can bind to many other compounds to create complexes. These complexes are constantly broken down throughout the gastrointestinal system into smaller and more easily absorbed molecules [30]. Approximately 50% of unbound pyrroline and penterosin may be retrieved in human urine. However, when consuming meals that include pentosein (impure substances), only 2% of the pentose is excreted in the urine [31]. Gaining insight into the metabolic process of AGEs in food indicates that minimising the consumption of AGEs from food can decrease the influx of AGEs into the human body and mitigate their detrimental effects on human health.

4.3 Dietary AGE contributes to type 1 diabetes mellitus

Recent studies have emphasised the significance of consuming dietary AGEs (dAGEs) as risk factors for the establishment of T1D. High levels of dAGEs in the bloodstream are a significant environmental risk factor for this variant of diabetes. When combined with the presence of autoantibodies, which is a recognised risk factor, high dAGE concentrations can place individuals at a higher risk of developing T1D [32]. Studies conducted on mice have indicated that dAGEs trigger malfunction in β-cells by binding to their receptor RAGE, which leads to oxidative stress and a shortfall in insulin production [33]. Research conducted on isolated islets has shown that long-term exposure to dAGEs decreases the amount of insulin present in the islets and reduces insulin secretion in response to glucose stimulation. Additionally, it leads to an increased infiltration of immune cells into the pancreatic islets. These effects are believed to be caused by the production of mitochondrial superoxide and a decrease in ATP production [33, 34]. High levels of dAGEs were also discovered to hinder the production of ATP, preventing the ATP-dependent opening of the potassium (K^+) channel, and resulting in decreased insulin release in response to glucose stimulation. dAGEs may also hinder the release of insulin by increasing the activity of nitric oxide synthase (NOS), leading to higher levels of nitric oxide in the pancreatic islets and INS cells (A rat cell line of mammalian origin that dAGE has the ability to store and release insulin in response to a broad spectrum of glucose concentrations). As a consequence, this led to the suppression of the cytochrome c oxidase, a key component of the electron transport chain, leading to a decrease in the production of ATP and a decrease in the release of insulin [34]. Problems with insulin secretion and the infiltration of islet cells were observed in healthy rats, even though they did not have diabetes [33]. Furthermore, mice that were fed a low AGE diet exhibited elevated levels of islet hormones such as insulin, proinsulin, and glucagon, and experienced less immune infiltration, in comparison to mice on a high AGE diet [35, 36]. An investigation conducted on humans revealed that children at risk of developing T1D who eventually developed the condition had greater levels of dAGEs in their blood serum compared to those who did not proceed to T1D [33]. This indicates that consuming higher levels of dAGEs might negatively affect the function of β-cells, which in turn can contribute to the development of T1D.

Additional research has demonstrated that the impact of dAGEs extends beyond the postnatal period and also influences the functioning of β-cells throughout the perinatal and prenatal stages. Studies have shown that the presence of dAGEs in the blood of mothers and the food consumed by infants might lead to an early increase in the levels of dAGEs in newborns' blood. This can affect their susceptibility to inflammatory disorders like T1D [37]. Research conducted on NOD mice models has shown that restricting the intake of dAGEs in mothers from conception to giving birth has a substantial impact on the fasting blood glucose levels and insulin responses to glucose in their offspring, leading to elevations in these parameters [35, 36]. In addition, pancreatic islets from the offspring mice whose mothers received high dAGE in diet during and after gestation exhibited a higher level of immune cell infiltration compared to the newborns whose mothers had a low dAGE [36]. The intergenerational dAGE research found a noteworthy decrease in the incidence of T1D in mice that were given a reduced dAGE diet compared to those fed a high dAGE diet [35]. In healthy persons, there is a direct correlation between the levels of dAGEs in the bloodstream and the production of insulin [38]. However, persons with T1D who have impairments in kidney or liver function typically see a significant reduction in the rate at which dAGEs are cleared from their bodies [39]. These changes affect insulin secretion and sensitivity. The higher occurrence of obesity in persons with T1D may also raise the probability of developing liver conditions such as non-alcoholic steatohepatitis (NASH) and non-alcoholic fatty liver disease (NAFLD), which can affect the clearance of dAGEs [40, 41]. Obesity is now being more widely acknowledged as being linked to an earlier onset of T1D and the development of a T1D-like condition characterised by immune infiltration and islet autoimmunity. Consuming less dAGEs through food increases insulin sensitivity in overweight persons and reduces chronic low-grade inflammation [42]. Food with high dAGE content has a negative effect on kidney function in overweight and obese people, as well as on liver function in animal models of obesity and liver fibrosis. Collectively, these studies indicate that elevated levels of dAGEs in the body might result in harm to β-cells and hinder their normal functioning. This may occur through the influence of immunoregulation, hence leading to the development of T1D.

4.4 Complications due to dAGEs in type 1 diabetes mellitus patients

The dAGEs have a substantial impact on the development of health issues in people diagnosed with T1D. T1D is predominantly an autoimmune condition characterised by the loss of pancreatic beta cells, resulting in a lack of insulin. AGEs, which are naturally formed in the body during metabolic processes, are typically controlled by several enzymes, as explained previously in this chapter. However, dAGEs are an additional group of these molecules that disrupt the optimal level of AGEs that the body is meant to uphold. Even in persons with good health, dAGEs' accumulation in addition to the pre-existing endogenous AGEs in the body may cause health issues. In individuals with T1D, there is a low production of insulin in the body, leading to poor absorption of glucose molecules from the blood. This puts those with the disorder at risk of having different health concerns. Elevated blood glucose levels might potentially lead to the production of AGEs within the body, resulting in an increased concentration of endogenous AGEs. In addition, the introduction of dAGEs increases the likelihood of problems that individuals with T1D are already susceptible to. Exogenous AGEs obtained from food sources, dAGEs, worsen several diabetes problems by causing oxidative stress, inflammation, and malfunction in cells.

These dAGEs frequently build up inside cells in several locations affected by diabetic problems, such as the kidney, retina, and atherosclerotic plaques. Protein glycation hinders normal protein activities by affecting molecular structure, modifying enzyme activity, decreasing breakdown ability, and impeding receptor recognition. Glycation affects cell functioning through several mechanisms, including the denaturation and functional deterioration of target proteins and lipids, the development of organ damage owing to the accumulation of AGEs in tissues, the activation of receptor-mediated signal pathways in cells, and the formation of oxidative stress and carbonyl stress. The formation of intermolecular collagen cross-links induced by dAGEs results in reduced compliance of arteries and myocardium increased vascular stiffness, and the development of diastolic dysfunction and systolic hypertension.

Autoantibodies against serum dAGEs can create AGE-immune complexes in diabetic individuals. The interaction between dAGEs and RAGE can activate the NF-Kβ pathway, resulting in inflammation. This inflammation can ultimately aggravate problems such as retinopathy, cataracts, nephropathy, neuropathy, cardiomyopathy, and more, which people suffering from T1D are already at risk.

4.4.1 Cardiovascular issue

dAGEs stimulate the generation of ROS in endothelial cells. This oxidative stress causes endothelial cell damage and impairs their function. They decrease the presence of NO, an essential molecule for widening blood vessels, resulting in the narrowing of blood vessels (vasoconstriction) and high blood pressure (hypertension). dAGEs stimulate the activation of NF-κB via interacting with RAGEs. NF-κB is a transcription factor that increases the expression of pro-inflammatory cytokines, including TNF-α, IL-6, and IL-1β. NF-κB activation triggers inflammatory cytokines that cause endothelial dysfunction and oxidative stress, resulting in a vicious cycle. These activities result in the dysfunction of endothelial cells, which is the initial stage of cardiovascular problems. dAGEs have a role in the process of oxidising low-density lipoprotein (LDL), resulting in the formation of oxidised LDL. Macrophages ingest this oxidised LDL, transforming into foam cells, which serve as the fundamental components of atherosclerotic plaques [43, 44]. In addition, dAGEs promote the growth and movement of vascular smooth muscle cells into the inner layer of blood arteries, leading to the thickening of the vascular walls and the development of atherosclerotic plaques. These molecules also enhance the production of matrix metalloproteases, which are enzymes responsible for breaking down the extracellular matrix. This deterioration results in the weakening of the fibrous cap of atherosclerotic plaques, rendering them more susceptible to rupture [45]. Atherosclerosis risk is heightened by lipid oxidation, proliferation of vascular smooth muscle, and destabilisation of the atherosclerotic plaque. dAGEs create cross-links with collagen in the vascular wall. This cross-linking causes a decrease in vascular flexibility, resulting in higher systolic blood pressure, which is a risk factor for cardiovascular disease [46]. They intensify the process of platelet activation and aggregation, hence promoting a condition that is prone to blood clot formation. This elevates the likelihood of thrombus development within the blood arteries [47]. dAGEs can also increase the production of tissue factors in endothelial cells and monocytes, which stimulates the coagulation cascade and further amplifies the creation of blood clots [48]. Also, they further contribute to myocardial fibrosis by encouraging the proliferation of fibroblasts and the creation of collagen in the heart. This fibrosis hinders the ability of the heart to function properly and can result in heart failure. These chemicals stimulate the enlargement of heart muscle cells, which is a compensatory reaction to heightened stiffness in blood vessels and high blood pressure. Over a period of time, this excessive growth of the heart muscle can result in the inability of the heart to effectively pump blood, which is known as heart failure [49]. All of the aforementioned processes ultimately contribute to the development of cardiovascular problems in individuals with T1D, particularly those with a high concentration of AGEs in their bodies.

4.4.2 Renal complications

dAGEs have a crucial impact on the progression and exacerbation of kidney problems, namely diabetic nephropathy, in people diagnosed with T1D. These molecules gather in the glomerular basement membrane, resulting in structural alterations and thickening, which is a characteristic feature of diabetic nephropathy. The thickening impairs the glomeruli's filtration function, resulting in a lower glomerular filtration rate and the onset of proteinuria. dAGEs further activate mesangial cells, prompting them to overproduce extracellular matrix proteins, resulting in the growth of mesangial cells and the development of glomerulosclerosis [50]. They stimulate the synthesis of cytokines including TGF-β and connective tissue growth factor, which enhance the proliferation of mesangial cells and the formation of extracellular matrix. These physiological alterations in the kidney may have an adverse effect on the glomerulus. dAGEs enhance the production of fibrogenic factors such as TGF-β, which stimulate fibroblasts to generate collagen and other components of the extracellular matrix. As a result, tubulointerstitial fibrosis occurs, which is marked by the buildup of extracellular matrix proteins in the interstitial area of the kidney, causing a decline in kidney function [51]. In addition, dAGEs stimulate the attraction and activation of macrophages and other inflammatory cells in the renal interstitium. The persistent inflammatory response exacerbates tissue damage and fibrosis, leading to a further decline in renal function [52]. dAGEs induce both structural and functional harm to podocytes, which are specialised cells essential for preserving the integrity of the glomerular filtration barrier. The injury causes the foot processes of the podocytes to become effaced, and detached from the glomerular basement membrane, and increases the permeability of the glomerulus, leading to the presence of protein in the urine (proteinuria). These substances cause programmed cell death in podocytes by increasing oxidative stress and activating signalling pathways that promote cell death. This leads to the loss of podocytes and worsens the function of the glomerular filtration barrier [53]. In addition to these factors, the production of oxidative stress by dAGEs, the reduction of bioavailability of NO leading to impairment of endothelial function, and the interaction between dAGEs and RAGE, which activates the NFKB pathway and triggers the release of inflammatory cytokines, collectively contribute to the impairment of renal functions in patients with T1D when there is a high concentration of dAGEs in their system.

4.4.3 Retinal complications

dAGEs induce changes in the structure and function of retinal tissues through several pathways, including oxidative stress, inflammation, and impaired blood vessel function. These changes might potentially result in retinal problems in individuals with T1D. These molecules build up in the basement membranes of retinal capillaries, resulting in their thickening and impairment of their usual function. This thickening exacerbates retinal ischaemia by lowering capillary permeability and reducing the quantity of oxygen and nutrients reaching the retinal tissues. dAGEs induce apoptosis of pericytes, which are contractile cells that surround endothelial cells in capillaries. Due to the loss of pericytes, the capillaries become unstable, resulting in the development of microaneurysms. Microaneurysms possess the capability to rupture, resulting in intra-retinal haemorrhages and contributing to the progression of diabetic retinopathy. dAGEs also cause the loss of retinal endothelial cells, leading to increased permeability of blood vessels and rupture of the blood-retinal barrier. This rupture allows fluid and proteins to enter the retinal tissue, leading to the formation of macular oedema, which severely impairs vision [54]. dAGEs stimulate the production of VEGF, leading to the formation of leaky new blood vessels. This process contributes to the development of macular oedema, which leads to visual impairment. dAGEs also stimulate the production of high quantities of VEGF, which stimulates the development of new blood vessels. Proliferative diabetic retinopathy refers to the growth of new blood vessels in the vitreous humour. These vessels tend to rupture, resulting in vitreous haemorrhage and the possibility of retinal detachment. In addition, these molecules stimulate Müller glial cells, which have a crucial function in preserving the performance of the retina, resulting in their impairment. Müller cells that have been activated emit pro-inflammatory cytokines, which worsen retinal damage by contributing to neuroinflammation [55]. Also, dAGEs further stimulate retinal astrocytes, leading to the disruption of the structural and functional integrity of the retinal blood-brain barrier. This activation exacerbates inflammation and leads to retinal damage, hence further compromising visual function. In addition to these factors, the presence of excessive. These molecules in individuals with T1D may lead to diabetic retinopathy through oxidative stress and activation of the NFKB pathway, resulting in the production of inflammatory cytokines [56, 57].

4.4.4 Neural complications

dAGEs destroy peripheral nerves directly, by oxidative stress and inflammation. This eventually results in demyelination and axonal decay. dAGEs also damage the microvasculature which in turn impairs circulation to the nerves, which then further contributes to neuropathic pain and sensation loss. And these physical problems lead to neurological issues down the road. Cross-linking of collagen due to dAGEs impairs the normal structure of the skin, making individuals more susceptible to infections and delaying wound healing. This leads to dAGE accumulation in bone collagen, which has a deleterious impact on bone quality and an increased fracture susceptibility. dAGEs induce stiffening of tendon and ligament collagens, resulting in restricted joint motion and diabetic neuroarthropathy (limited joint mobility syndrome). dAGEs inhibit keratinocytes and fibroblasts, which are responsible for the proper turnover of cells while healing wounds. This results in wound healing deficits and predisposes to the development of chronic ulcers in particular on the lower extremities. dAGEs are likely to participate in autonomic neuropathy of the gut manifesting as gastroparesis (altered gastric emptying). A condition that includes nausea, vomiting, and bloating which makes diabetes management more complex.

In addition, other complications from dAGEs in type 1 diabetes mellitus patients, may have complications in skin, bone joint, gastrointestinal and wound healing.

5. Mitigation strategies for dietary AGEs in type 1 diabetes

Advanced glycation end products (AGEs) are a significant trigger of the complications in type 1 diabetes. These include complications of diabetes mellitus such as diabetic retinopathy, nephropathy, and cardiovascular diseases. Perhaps worst of all, these issues are even more severe when dietary AGEs—which you ingest from food instead of forming in your body—come into play. In turn, these adverse effects can be alleviated by implementing dietary strategies that minimise ingestion of AGEs.

5.1 Cooking methods

5.1.1 Low-temperature cooking

Boiling, simmering (not boiling; only slightly bubbling) poaching, and steaming are better options than using high temperatures for cooking such as grilling, frying, or roasting. These methods reduce the formation of AGEs in foods. For example, boiled chicken will have MUCH less AGE production compared to grilling or broiling it [56].

5.1.2 Use of acidic marinades

Prior to cooking, marinating meals in acidic solutions such as lemon juice, vinegar, or wine helps reduce the production of advanced glycation end products (AGEs). The presence of acidity hinders the Maillard reaction, which is the process responsible for the development of AGEs [57].

5.2 Dietary choices

5.2.1 Increase consumption of fresh foods

Unprocessed fruits and vegetables have lower amounts of dAGEs in comparison to processed foods and those that are cooked at high temperatures. This is because of their elevated water content and reduced levels of protein and fat, which serve as substrates for the development of dAGEs during the cooking process. These foods are rich in antioxidants, including vitamins C and E, flavonoids, and polyphenols. Antioxidants have a vital function in counteracting free radicals and diminishing oxidative stress, which is intensified by dAGEs. For example, incorporating fruits like berries and citrus fruits, as well as greens like spinach, broccoli, and kale into one's diet can assist in reducing oxidative damage. A multitude of fruits and vegetables exhibit anti-inflammatory characteristics. For instance, the presence of flavonoids in apples and onions, as well as carotenoids in carrots and sweet potatoes, can effectively decrease inflammation associated with the buildup of dAGEs and the resulting problems in diabetes. Whole grains, such as oats, brown rice, quinoa, and barley, naturally have low levels of dAGEs, particularly when prepared using low-temperature cooking techniques such as boiling or steaming. This aids in reducing the consumption of detrimental dAGEs. The dietary fibre included in whole grains helps to regulate blood glucose levels and enhance insulin sensitivity. Enhanced regulation of blood sugar levels decreases the creation of naturally occurring AGEs, as high blood sugar levels play a significant role in the synthesis of AGEs in the body. Whole grains provide a significant amount of vital minerals such as B vitamins, magnesium, and zinc. These nutrients are beneficial for maintaining general metabolic health and can help lower the risk of issues associated with high levels of dAGEs [56, 57].

5.2.2 Limit processed foods

Processed foods, such as pre-cooked and packaged meals, may include elevated amounts of dAGEs as a result of cooking methods involving high temperatures. This process, known as the Maillard reaction, happens when amino acids and reducing sugars undergo a chemical reaction to produce both food taste and colour. However, consuming significant quantities of these reaction products can be hazardous. Sausage, bacon, hot dogs, and deli cuts are rich in advanced glycation end products (AGEs). Similarly, this applies to baked foods such as cakes. The items mentioned include cookies, pastries, bread, packaged snacks such as chips and crackers, ready-to-eat meals commonly seen at fast food restaurants, canned soups, and frozen entrees. These meals, which are also high in fats and proteins, have the potential to generate dAGEs when they undergo processing and cooking.

5.3 Nutritional interventions

5.3.1 Supplements

Omega-3 fatty acids, vitamins C and E, and alpha-lipoic acid are examples of dietary supplements that include antioxidant qualities that can assist in mitigating the oxidative stress that is caused by dAGEs. It has been investigated whether or not aminoguanidine has the ability to prevent the production of dAGEs; nevertheless, due to the fact that more investigation is required, its implementation is not yet frequently recommended [56].

5.3.2 Glyoxalase 1 inducers

Compounds that stimulate glyoxalase 1, an enzyme that is responsible for the detoxification of dAGE may help in reducing circulating dAGEs in the human body. Some polyphenols, such as those found in green tea and berries, are examples of such substances [56].

5.4 Lifestyle modifications

5.4.1 Regular physical activity

Engaging in regular physical exercise can lower the presence of dAGEs by employing many methods, all of which contribute to enhanced metabolic well-being and reduced dAGE buildup. It improves the body's ability to respond to insulin, leading to better control of blood glucose levels. Exercise promotes glucose absorption in muscle cells without relying on insulin by activating AMP-activated protein kinase (AMPK) and moving GLUT4 glucose transporters to the cell membrane. Also, it enhances the body's natural antioxidant defence, which includes increasing the activities of superoxide dismutase, catalase, and glutathione peroxidase. Increased antioxidant capacity aids in counteracting ROS, hence diminishing oxidative stress and circulating dAGEs. Exercise exerts anti-inflammatory effects, hence reducing chronic inflammation linked to elevated levels of dAGEs. It also reduces pro-inflammatory cytokines, such as TNF-α and IL-6, which play a role in the inflammatory pathways that lead to dAGE-related damage. Physical activity stimulates the secretion of nitric oxide (NO) from the cells lining the blood vessels, known as endothelial cells. This leads to enhanced circulation and a decreased likelihood of cardiovascular problems associated with dAGE and T1D. Exercise can improve the elimination of dAGEs by promoting better kidney function and higher excretion through urine. Enhanced renal function facilitates the more effective elimination of dAGEs from the circulatory system, hence diminishing their buildup in bodily tissues [58].

5.4.2 Hydration

It helps kidneys filter blood and reduce tissue dAGE buildup. Increased urine flow reduces AGEs and their precursors. Hydration helps maintain blood volume, decrease blood glucose, improve insulin sensitivity, and preserve cellular function. Preventing dAGE formation and oxidative stress requires antioxidant and free radical equilibrium [59].

5.4.3 Reduce stress

Stress affects AGE production and accumulation of dAGE through physiological and biochemical mechanisms. Chronic stress increases oxidative stress, inflammation, and AGEs both eAGEs and dAGEs. Mindfulness, meditation, yoga, and deep breathing boost antioxidant defences and reduce oxidative stress. Stress management increases antioxidant enzyme activity, neutralises ROS, and reduces dAGE-damaging inflammatory indicators. Regular exercise improves insulin action and glucose absorption, reducing AGE risk. Healthy immune systems can combat dAGE damage. Stress can also motivate healthy eating and exercise.

6. Conclusion

AGE molecules are unavoidable. These are entities that are produced in our body (endogenous AGE) and are present in our food (dietary AGE). They are present when the cells of our body carry out metabolic activities and when we prepare food in our kitchen. It is present in small or large quantities in almost all food items that are cooked. The body has a mechanism for clearing it from the system, but, recent lifestyle choices have stretched the body's capacity of mitigating this class of chemicals beyond its limits. Processed food, high-sugar content, food cooked at high temperatures, etc. are very high in these substances which are responsible for various lifestyle diseases. Type 1 diabetes mellitus, which was earlier considered an autoimmune disorder, is now known to be one of the diseases that can be caused by this chemical. Although dietary AGEs are not different from the endogenous AGEs formed in the body, the increase of dAGEs in the system overwhelms the enzymatic pathways and an excess of these molecules begins to accumulate in our body. These accumulated dAGEs can cause inflammation in different cells of the body, including the β-Cells of pancreatic islets, therefore causing hindrance in insulin formation. This may be one of the environmental causes of T1D in present times. Moreover, when it comes to people who are already suffering from diabetes, they already have a high concentration of glucose in their blood and their insulin production system is already impaired. In such cases, the body is already vulnerable to various diseases like, cardiomyopathy, diabetic neuropathy, nephropathy, retinopathy, etc. This is because the high glucose content in the blood easily undergoes the Maillard reaction and forms AGEs with proteins on the surface of many cell surfaces, especially collagen. For patients like this, there is already the presence of an above-average concentration of dAGEs in their bodies. Introducing further AGEs into the system through the diet may accelerate diabetes associated conditions which these patients are already vulnerable to. Therefore, patients with type 1 diabetes mellitus should be very careful and avoid foods that are high in dAGEs and increase antioxidants in their system, which will help reduce the concentration of already existing AGEs in the body.

Conflict of interest

The authors declare that there are no conflicts of interest regarding the publication of this chapter.

Acronyms and abbreviations

AGE	advanced glycation end products
AGER	AGE-specific receptor
CML	carboxymethyl lysine
dAGE	dietary advanced glycation end-products
GTP	guanosine triphosphate
HLA	human leukocyte antigens
IL	interleukin
JAK	Janus kinase activators of transcription
LDL	low-density lipoprotein
MAPK	mitogen-activated protein kinase
MG-H1	methyl-glyoxal derived hydroimidazolones
MHC	multihistocompatibility protein
MSR	macrophage scavenger receptors
NAFLD	non-alcoholic fatty liver disease
NASH	non-alcoholic steatohepatitis
NF-κB	nuclear factor kappa B
PI3K	phosphoinositide 3-kinase
RAGE	receptor for advanced glycation end products
ROS	reactive oxygen species
SOD	superoxide dismutase
STAT	signal transducers and activators of transcription
T1D	type 1 diabetes mellitus
TGFβ	transforming growth factor beta
TNF-α	tumour necrosis factor-α
VEGF	vascular endothelial growth factor
ATP	adenosine triphosphate

Author details

Sanchari Bhattacharyya[1] and Sagar Acharya[2*]

1 Centre for Life Sciences, Vidyasagar University, Midnapore, West Bengal, India

2 Department of Zoology, Vidyasagar University, Midnapore, West Bengal, India

*Address all correspondence to: sagar.gene@gmail.com

References

[1] Wang Z, Xie Z, Lu Q, Chang C, Zhou Z. Beyond genetics: What causes type 1 diabetes. Clinical Reviews in Allergy and Immunology. 2017;**52**:273-286. DOI: 10.1007/s12016-016-8592-1

[2] Maahs DM, West NA, Lawrence JM, Mayer-Davis EJ. Epidemiology of type 1 diabetes. Endocrinology and Metabolism Clinics of North America. 2010;**39**:481-497. DOI: 10.1016/j.ecl.2010.05.011

[3] Prasad C, Davis KE, Imrhan V, Juma S, Vijayagopal P. Advanced glycation end products and risks for chronic diseases: Intervening through lifestyle modification. American Journal of Lifestyle Medicine. 2019;**13**:384-404. DOI: 10.1177/1559827617708991

[4] Bloemer J, Bhattacharya S, Amin R, Suppiramaniam V. Impaired Insulin Signaling and Mechanisms of Memory Loss. Progress in molecular biology and translational science; 2014. pp. 413-449. DOI: 10.1016/B978-0-12-800101-1.00013-2

[5] Liu S, Sun H, Ma G, Zhang T, Wang L, Pei H, et al. Insights into flavor and key influencing factors of Maillard reaction products: A recent update. Frontiers in Nutrition. 2022;**9**:973677. DOI: 10.3389/fnut.2022.973677

[6] Mengstie MA, Chekol Abebe E, Behaile Teklemariam A, Tilahun Mulu A, Agidew MM, Teshome Azezew M, et al. Endogenous advanced glycation end products in the pathogenesis of chronic diabetic complications. Frontiers in Molecular Biosciences. 2022;**9**:1002710. DOI: 10.3389/fmolb.2022.1002710

[7] Khalid M, Petroianu G, Adem A. Advanced glycation end products and diabetes mellitus: Mechanisms and perspectives. Biomolecules. 2022;**12**:542. DOI: 10.3390/biom12040542

[8] Hollenbach M, Zipprich A. The role of glyoxalase-I in oxidant stress of liver damage. In: The Liver. Elsevier, Academic Press; 2018. pp. 71-78. DOI: 10.1016/B978-0-12-803951-9.00007-0

[9] Yadav N, Palkhede JD, Kim S-Y. Anti-glucotoxicity effect of phytoconstituents via inhibiting MGO-AGEs formation and breaking MGO-AGEs. International Journal of Molecular Sciences. 2023;**24**:7672. DOI: 10.3390/ijms24087672

[10] Perrone A, Giovino A, Benny J, Martinelli F. Advanced glycation end products (AGEs): Biochemistry, signaling, analytical methods, and epigenetic effects. Oxidative Medicine and Cellular Longevity. 2020;**2020**:1-18. DOI: 10.1155/2020/3818196

[11] Fotheringham AK, Gallo LA, Borg DJ, Forbes JM. Advanced glycation end products (AGEs) and chronic kidney disease: Does the modern diet AGE the kidney? Nutrients. 2022;**14**:2675. DOI: 10.3390/nu14132675

[12] Chen J-H, Lin X, Bu C, Zhang X. Role of advanced glycation end products in mobility and considerations in possible dietary and nutritional intervention strategies. Nutrition & Metabolism (London). 2018;**15**:72. DOI: 10.1186/s12986-018-0306-7

[13] Jia W, Guo A, Zhang R, Shi L. Mechanism of natural antioxidants regulating advanced glycosylation end products of Maillard reaction. Food Chemistry. 2023;**404**:134541. DOI: 10.1016/J.FOODCHEM.2022.134541

[14] Gutowska K, Czajkowski K, Kuryłowicz A. Receptor for the advanced glycation end products (RAGE) pathway in adipose tissue metabolism. International Journal of Molecular Sciences. 2023;**24**:10982. DOI: 10.3390/ijms241310982

[15] Carr KD, Weiner SP, Vasquez C, Schmidt AM. Involvement of the Receptor for Advanced Glycation End Products (RAGE) in high fat-high sugar diet-induced anhedonia in rats. Physiology & Behavior. 2023;**271**:114337. DOI: 10.1016/j.physbeh.2023.114337

[16] Kim CH, Kang H-Y, Kim G, Park J, Nam BY, Park JT, et al. Soluble receptors for advanced glycation end-products prevent unilateral ureteral obstruction-induced renal fibrosis. Frontiers in Pharmacology. 2023;**14**:1172269. DOI: 10.3389/fphar.2023.1172269

[17] Aradillas-García C, Vega-Cárdenas M, Vargas-Morales JM, Portales-Pérez DP, Gómez-Ojeda A, Luevano-Contreras C. Soluble receptor for advanced glycation end-products (sRAGE) in childhood obesity: Association with gene expression of RAGE and cardiometabolic markers. Nutrición Hospitalaria. 2023;**40**(5):960-966. DOI: 10.20960/nh.04666

[18] Lin J, Tang Y, Kang Q, Chen A. Curcumin eliminates the inhibitory effect of advanced glycation end-products (AGEs) on gene expression of AGE receptor-1 in hepatic stellate cells in vitro. Laboratory Investigation. 2012;**92**:827-841. DOI: 10.1038/labinvest.2012.53

[19] Gong Y, Liu Z, Zhang Y, Zhang J, Zheng Y, Wu Z. AGER1 deficiency-triggered ferroptosis drives fibrosis progression in nonalcoholic steatohepatitis with type 2 diabetes mellitus. Cell Death Discovery. 2023;**9**:178. DOI: 10.1038/s41420-023-01477-z

[20] Sowndhar Rajan B, Krishnan K, Vellaichamy E. Diet-derived advanced glycation end products (dAGEs) induce proinflammatory cytokine expression in cardiac and renal tissues of experimental mice: Protective effect of curcumin. Cardiovascular Toxicology. 2022;**22**:35-51. DOI: 10.1007/s12012-021-09697-4

[21] Gutierrez-Mariscal FM, Cardelo MP, de la Cruz S, Alcala-Diaz JF, Roncero-Ramos I, Guler I, et al. Reduction in circulating advanced glycation end products by mediterranean diet is associated with increased likelihood of type 2 diabetes remission in patients with coronary heart disease: From the cordioprev study. Molecular Nutrition & Food Research. 2021;**65**(1):1901290. DOI: 10.1002/mnfr.201901290

[22] Sessa L, Gatti E, Zeni F, Antonelli A, Catucci A, Koch M, et al. The receptor for advanced glycation end-products (RAGE) is only present in mammals, and belongs to a family of cell adhesion molecules (CAMs). PLoS ONE. 2014;**9**:e86903. DOI: 10.1371/journal.pone.0086903

[23] Senatus LM, Schmidt AM. The AGE-RAGE axis: Implications for age-associated arterial diseases. Frontiers in Genetics. 2017;**8**. DOI: 10.3389/fgene.2017.00187

[24] Twarda-Clapa A, Olczak A, Białkowska AM, Koziołkiewicz M. Advanced glycation end-products (AGEs): Formation, chemistry, classification, receptors, and diseases related to AGEs. Cells. 2022;**11**:1312. DOI: 10.3390/cells11081312

[25] Rouhiainen A, Kuja-Panula J, Tumova S, Rauvala H. RAGE-Mediated Cell Signaling. Methods in

Molecular Biology. 2013. pp. 239-263. DOI: 10.1007/978-1-62703-230-8_15

[26] Uribarri J, Cai W, Peppa M, Goodman S, Ferrucci L, Striker G, et al. Circulating glycotoxins and dietary advanced glycation endproducts: Two links to inflammatory response, oxidative stress, and aging. The Journals of Gerontology. Series A, Biological Sciences and Medical Sciences. 2007;**62**:427-433. DOI: 10.1093/gerona/62.4.427

[27] Lander HM, Tauras JM, Ogiste JS, Hori O, Moss RA, Schmidt AM. Activation of the receptor for advanced glycation end products triggers a p21-dependent mitogen-activated protein kinase pathway regulated by oxidant stress. Journal of Biological Chemistry. 1997;**272**:17810-17814. DOI: 10.1074/jbc.272.28.17810

[28] Zheng W, Li H, Go Y, Chan XH(F), Huang Q, Wu J. Research advances on the damage mechanism of skin glycation and related inhibitors. Nutrients. 2022;**14**:4588. DOI: 10.3390/nu14214588

[29] He C, Sabol J, Mitsuhashi T, Vlassara H. Dietary glycotoxins: Inhibition of reactive products by aminoguanidine facilitates renal clearance and reduces tissue sequestration. Diabetes. 1999;**48**:1308-1315. DOI: 10.2337/diabetes.48.6.1308

[30] Förster A, Kühne Y, Henle TO. Studies on absorption and elimination of dietary Maillard reaction products. Annals of the New York Academy of Sciences. 2005;**1043**:474-481. DOI: 10.1196/annals.1333.054

[31] Peppa M, Mavroeidi I. Experimental animal studies support the role of dietary advanced glycation end products in health and disease. Nutrients. 2021;**13**:3467. DOI: 10.3390/nu13103467

[32] Beyan H, Riese H, Hawa MI, Beretta G, Davidson HW, Hutton JC, et al. Glycotoxin and autoantibodies are additive environmentally determined predictors of type 1 diabetes. Diabetes. 2012;**61**:1192-1198. DOI: 10.2337/db11-0971

[33] Coughlan MT, Yap FYT, Tong DCK, Andrikopoulos S, Gasser A, Thallas-Bonke V, et al. Advanced glycation end products are direct modulators of β-cell function. Diabetes. 2011;**60**:2523-2532. DOI: 10.2337/db10-1033

[34] Zhao Z, Zhao C, Zhang XH, Zheng F, Cai W, Vlassara H, et al. Advanced glycation end products inhibit glucose-stimulated insulin secretion through nitric oxide-dependent inhibition of cytochrome c oxidase and adenosine triphosphate synthesis. Endocrinology. 2009;**150**:2569-2576. DOI: 10.1210/en.2008-1342

[35] Peppa M, He C, Hattori M, McEvoy R, Zheng F, Vlassara H. Fetal or neonatal low-glycotoxin environment prevents autoimmune diabetes in NOD mice. Diabetes. 2003;**52**:1441-1448. DOI: 10.2337/diabetes.52.6.1441

[36] Borg DJ, Yap FYT, Keshvari S, Simmons DG, Gallo LA, Fotheringham AK, et al. Perinatal exposure to high dietary advanced glycation end products in transgenic NOD8.3 mice leads to pancreatic beta cell dysfunction. Islets. 2018;**10**:10-24. DOI: 10.1080/19382014.2017.1405189

[37] Mericq V, Piccardo C, Cai W, Chen X, Zhu L, Striker GE, et al. Maternally transmitted and food-derived glycotoxins. Diabetes Care. 2010;**33**:2232-2237. DOI: 10.2337/dc10-1058

[38] Forbes JM, Sourris KC, de Courten MPJ, Dougherty SL, Chand V, Lyons JG, et al. Advanced glycation

end products (AGEs) are cross-sectionally associated with insulin secretion in healthy subjects. Amino Acids. 2014;**46**:321-326. DOI: 10.1007/s00726-013-1542-9

[39] Vlassara H, Uribarri J. Advanced glycation end products (AGE) and diabetes: Cause, effect, or both? Current Diabetes Reports. 2014;**14**:453. DOI: 10.1007/s11892-013-0453-1

[40] Barros B, Conte Santos D, Haas Pizarro M, Melo L, Brito GM. Type 1 diabetes and non-alcoholic fatty liver disease: When should we be concerned? A Nationwide Study in Brazil. Nutrients. 2017;**9**:878. DOI: 10.3390/nu9080878

[41] Bhatt HB, Smith RJ. Fatty liver disease in diabetes mellitus. Hepatobiliary Surgery and Nutrition. 2015;**4**:101-108. DOI: 10.3978/j.issn.2304-3881.2015.01.03

[42] De Courten B, De Courten MPJ, Soldatos G, Dougherty SL, Straznicky N, Schlaich M, et al. Diet low in advanced glycation end products increases insulin sensitivity in healthy overweight individuals: A double-blind, randomized, crossover trial. The American Journal of Clinical Nutrition. 2016;**103**:1426-1433. DOI: 10.3945/AJCN.115.125427

[43] Basta G. Advanced glycation end products and vascular inflammation: Implications for accelerated atherosclerosis in diabetes. Cardiovascular Research. 2004;**63**:582-592. DOI: 10.1016/j.cardiores.2004.05.001

[44] Schalkwijk CG, Stehouwer CDA. Vascular complications in diabetes mellitus: The role of endothelial dysfunction. Clinical Science. 2005;**109**:143-159. DOI: 10.1042/CS20050025

[45] Gong C, Qi Y, Xu Y, Tang X, Liang F, Chen L. Parecoxib improves atherosclerotic plaque stability by suppressing inflammation and inhibiting matrix metalloproteinases production. Biomedicine & Pharmacotherapy. 2021;**138**:111423. DOI: 10.1016/j.biopha.2021.111423

[46] Aronson D. Cross-linking of glycated collagen in the pathogenesis of arterial and myocardial stiffening of aging and diabetes. Journal of Hypertension. 2003;**21**:3-12. DOI: 10.1097/00004872-200301000-00002

[47] Kosmopoulos M, Drekolias D, Zavras PD, Piperi C, Papavassiliou AG. Impact of advanced glycation end products (AGEs) signaling in coronary artery disease. Biochimica et Biophysica Acta (BBA) - Molecular Basis of Disease. 2019;**1865**:611-619. DOI: 10.1016/j.bbadis.2019.01.006

[48] Stirban A, Gawlowski T, Roden M. Vascular effects of advanced glycation endproducts: Clinical effects and molecular mechanisms. Molecular Metabolism. 2014;**3**:94-108. DOI: 10.1016/j.molmet.2013.11.006

[49] Cheng Y, Wang Y, Yin R, Xu Y, Zhang L, Zhang Y, et al. Central role of cardiac fibroblasts in myocardial fibrosis of diabetic cardiomyopathy. Frontiers in Endocrinology (Lausanne). 2023;**14**:1162754. DOI: 10.3389/fendo.2023.1162754

[50] Zhang L, Wen P, Zhang J, Xia C, Xu J, Xu H, et al. Effects of exogenous advanced glycation end products on oxidative stress and renal injury in healthy mice. eFood. 2023;**4**:e105. DOI: 10.1002/efd2.105

[51] Ren LL, Li XJ, Duan TT, Li ZH, Yang JZ, Zhang YM, et al. Transforming growth factor-β signaling: From tissue fibrosis to therapeutic opportunities. Chemico-Biological Interactions.

2023;**369**:110289. DOI: 10.1016/J.CBI.2022.110289

[52] Garay-Sevilla ME, Rojas A, Portero-Otin M, Uribarri J. Dietary AGEs as exogenous boosters of inflammation. Nutrients. 2021;**13**:2802. DOI: 10.3390/nu13082802

[53] Bettiga A, Fiorio F, Di Marco F, Trevisani F, Romani A, Porrini E, et al. The modern Western diet rich in advanced glycation end-products (AGEs): An overview of its impact on obesity and early progression of renal pathology. Nutrients. 2019;**11**:1748. DOI: 10.3390/nu11081748

[54] Vlassara H, Striker GE. Advanced glycation endproducts in diabetes and diabetic complications. Endocrinology and Metabolism Clinics of North America. 2013;**42**:697-719. DOI: 10.1016/j.ecl.2013.07.005

[55] McDowell RE, Barabas P, Augustine J, Chevallier O, McCarron P, Chen M, et al. Müller glial dysfunction during diabetic retinopathy in rats is reduced by the acrolein-scavenging drug, 2-hydrazino-4,6-dimethylpyrimidine. Diabetologia. 2018;**61**:2654-2667. DOI: 10.1007/s00125-018-4707-y

[56] Milne R, Brownstein S. Advanced glycation end products and diabetic retinopathy. Amino Acids. 2013;**44**:1397-1407. DOI: 10.1007/s00726-011-1071-3

[57] Hadzi-Petrushev N, Angelovski M, Mladenov M. Advanced Glycation End Products and Diabetes. Obesity, Diabetes and Inflammation Contemporary Endocrinology. 2023. pp. 99-127. DOI: 10.1007/978-3-031-39721-9_5

[58] Alyafei A. The influence of regular physical exercise on the advanced glycated end products. Research International Journal of Community Medicine and Public Health. 2020;**1**:047-053. DOI: 10.37179/rijcmph.000009

[59] Dozio E, Caldiroli L, Molinari P, Castellano G, Delfrate NW, Romanelli MMC, et al. Accelerated AGEing: The impact of advanced glycation end products on the prognosis of chronic kidney disease. Antioxidants. 2023;**12**:584. DOI: 10.3390/antiox12030584

Chapter 7

The Relationships between the Biochemical Processes of Diabetes and Urinary and Genital Tract Alterations

Oluwafemi Adeleke Ojo, Tenifayo Soyinka,
Emmanuel Henry Ezenabor and Adebola Busola Ojo

Abstract

This abstract examines the complex interactions that occur between the metabolic processes linked to diabetes and the resulting changes in the genital and urinary tracts. Diabetes mellitus is a metabolic disease that affects several physiological systems, including the genital and urinary systems. Changes in the structure and function of the genitourinary system are a result of the complex network of biochemical pathways affected by diabetes. This thorough analysis explored the molecular pathways that connect diabetes to changes in renal function, urinary tract infections, and reproductive health. Comprehending these complex interactions is essential to the development of focused therapies aimed at reducing the negative effects of diabetes on the genital and urinary tracts and eventually enhancing the quality of life for those afflicted with this common metabolic disease.

Keywords: diabetes mellitus, urinary tract infections, genitourinary alterations, renal function, reproductive health

1. Introduction

Diabetes mellitus (DM) is caused by insufficient regulation of blood glucose levels [1]. Diabetes is a chronic metabolic condition characterized by elevated levels of glucose (sugar) in the bloodstream. Over an extended period, diabetes can lead to significant harm to the heart, blood vessels, eyes, kidneys, and nerves [2].

There are two major types of diabetes: type 1 diabetes and type 2 diabetes. Type 1 diabetes is an endocrine condition caused by pancreatic β cells ceasing to generate insulin, usually as a result of autoimmune damage, while type 2 diabetes is somewhat influenced and caused by genetic predisposition, a poor diet, and a sedentary lifestyle. The predisposition to genital infections and urinary tract infections (UTIs) in type 2 diabetes mellitus patients is a result of several factors, such as glucosuria,

IntechOpen

adherence of bacteria to the uroepithelium, and immune dysfunction. In addition to these major types, gestational diabetes, which occurs due to abnormal glucose tolerance that begins or is first detected during pregnancy, has been referred to as gestational diabetes mellitus (GDM) [3]. Glycolysis, gluconeogenesis, glycogenesis, and glycogenolysis are important biochemical metabolic pathways that regulate blood glucose levels, and the glucokinase (GK) enzyme plays a key role in glucose homeostasis. Any element, such as diabetes, that disrupts metabolic processes is harmful. The uptake of glucose by muscle, adipose tissue, liver, and brain is stimulated by glucose at physiological concentrations because β-cells are stimulated to synthesize and release insulin, which in turn inhibits hepatic gluconeogenesis and stimulates glycogen, protein synthesis, and lipogenesis while inhibiting lipolysis [4].

2. Prevalence and pathophysiology of diabetes mellitus

The incidence of type 2 diabetes has steadily increased over the past few decades, which has led to a notable increase in the prevalence of diabetes mellitus (DM). Based on data from the World Health Organization, there were more than 422 million adults worldwide who had diabetes mellitus in 2014, and it is anticipated that this number will continue to increase. Currently, approximately 537 million adults between the ages of 20 and 79 years have diabetes. By 2030 and 2045, this number is expected to increase to 643 million and 783 million, respectively [5].

Diabetes often results from hyperglycemia (which refers to high glucose in blood) and related metabolic disorders of fat, protein, and carbohydrate metabolism, which impact several human organs and impair their normal operation. The abnormal effects of hyperglycemia and related metabolic abnormalities on the normal structure and function of the microvasculature and macrovasculature, which form the basis of organ structure and function throughout the body, are primarily responsible for these disruptions, which occur gradually. Microvascular and macrovascular problems are caused by structural and functional abnormalities in the vasculature of organ systems [6].

3. Biochemical processes and changes in diabetes patients

3.1 Insulin production and regulation

The process of producing insulin involves several distinct stages. To enable the newly generated preproinsulin to enter the rough endoplasmic reticulum (RER) lumen and aid in the appropriate folding of proinsulin, which is stabilized by three disulfide bonds, a preproinsulin precursor must first be translated. This precursor contains an N-terminal signal sequence. Proinsulin is created by quick, probably cotranslational, cleavage of the preproinsulin signal peptide. Following its trafficking from the RER through the Golgi apparatus continuum, proinsulin (the first prohormone to be identified) is concentrated in specific areas of the trans-Golgi network at the locations where immature insulin granules develop. Here, two Ca2+-sensitive prohormone convertases initiate the conversion of proinsulin to insulin and C-peptide using carboxypeptidase's basic amino acid trimming of split-proinsulin intermediates. The ideal pH is acidic, and the entry of Ca2+ into a developing β-granule starts the synthesis of proinsulin, preventing insulin from building up outside of the organelle that stores it. Des-31,32-proinsulin makes up the majority of hyperproinsulinemia that is observed to be circulating in type 2 diabetes, which is indicative of the sequential processing of proinsulin [7].

Insulin deficiency inhibits glucose from entering insulin-sensitive cells in tissues such as the liver, muscles, and fat and from being properly metabolized. The organism increases the release of four counterregulatory hormones—glucagon, cortisol, growth hormone, and catecholamines—in response to intracellular glucopenia. Together, these hormones promote glucose synthesis through gluconeogenesis and glycogen breakdown; trigger lipolysis and ketogenesis; and cause hyperglycemia, osmotic polyuria, dehydration, increased thirst, and acidosis due to the buildup of ketoacids, primarily β-hydroxybutyrate (B-OHB), which surpass buffering capacity. Additionally, the resulting dehydration and restricted tissue perfusion cause lactic acidosis. Therefore, the signs and symptoms include polyuria, polydipsia, dehydration, tachycardia, deep sighing breathing (Kussmaul breathing), the smell of acetone on the breath, and nausea and abdominal pain that mimic an acute abdominal condition. Ironically, blood pressure can be normal or elevated due to catecholamine effects, even in cases of dehydration [8]. Persistent hyperglycemia results in oxidative stress, which damages β-cell function and decreases peripheral organ sensitivity to insulin [9]. Even in fed states, insulin is unable to limit hepatic gluconeogenesis in people with impaired insulin signaling, such as insulin resistance in type 2 diabetes; therefore, understanding these insulin-moderated pathways is essential for treatment goals [10].

3.2 Glucose metabolism and utilization

Through gluconeogenesis, glucose consumption, and glucose reabsorption from the renal glomerular filtrate, the kidney contributes significantly to glucose homeostasis. Approximately 20–25% of the glucose that is released into the bloodstream following an overnight fast comes from the kidneys through a process called gluconeogenesis. Under these postabsorptive conditions, the kidneys use approximately 10% of the body's total glucose. Renal gluconeogenesis increases in the postprandial phase following glucose administration and contributes to approximately 60% of endogenous glucose release. Nearly all of the 180 g of glucose that the kidneys filter daily is reabsorbed into the bloodstream. In both the postprandial and fasting stages, patients with type 2 diabetes have enhanced renal glucose absorption and release. Furthermore, the plasma glucose levels that typically cause glucosuria in healthy individuals do not cause glucosuria in these patients [11]. Hyperglycemia in individuals with non-insulin-dependent diabetic metabolic disease (NIDDM) is primarily caused by inadequate inhibition of endogenous glucose synthesis; nevertheless, subsequent glucose utilization differs little from postabsorptive glucose metabolism [12].

3.3 Roles of hormones and enzymes in diabetes

Hormones are biological coordinators that regulate the physiological activities of tissues through metabolic regulation; deviations from normal hormone concentrations result in pathological conditions such as diabetes [13]. Glucagon plays a crucial role in the onset and development of diabetes. Hyperglucagonemia is a common feature of all forms of diabetes in both humans and animals, suggesting that excess

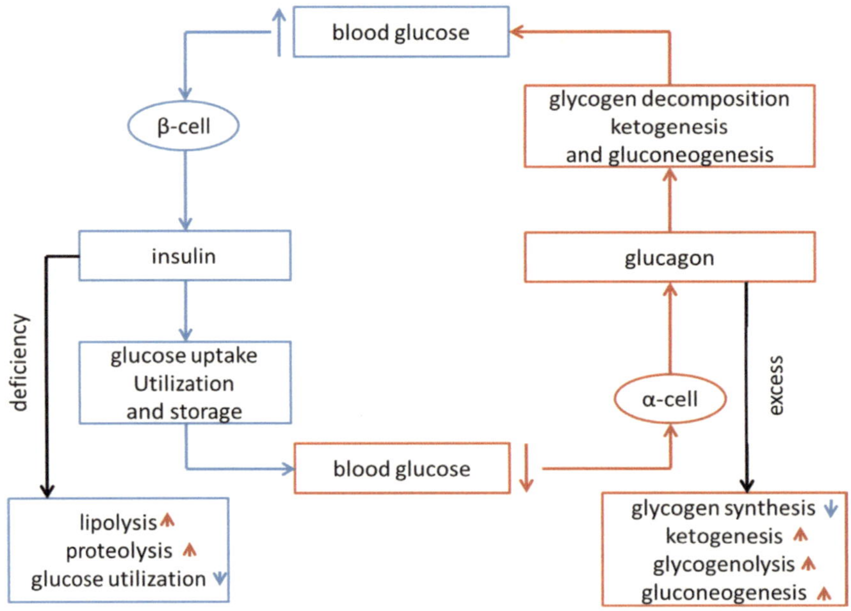

Figure 1.
Role of glucagon and insulin and its receptor in the pathogenesis of diabetes.

glucagon is more important for the onset of diabetes than insufficient insulin is. Recent research has shown that glucagon and glucagon receptor (GCGR) blockade can alleviate hyperglycemia in both humans and animals, demonstrating the critical roles that glucagon and GCGR play in the etiology of diabetes (**Figure 1**) [14].

4. Urinary tract alterations in diabetes patients

4.1 Diabetic bladder dysfunction (DBD)/diabetic nephropathy

Diabetic bladder dysfunction refers to the problems that occur in the bladder of diabetic mellitus patients. In the early phases of diabetes polyuria, hyperglycemia-induced polyuria plays a significant pathophysiological role, leading to compensatory bladder hypertrophy and related myogenic and neurogenic changes. Patients with urine voiding difficulties experience the usual signs and symptoms of diabetic cystopathy (hypocontractile detrusor or atonic bladder) as a result of the buildup of toxic metabolites and the subsequent decompensation of bladder tissue and function. Participating factors include neuronal damage, urothelial malfunction, and changes in the physiology of the detrusor muscle.

Glucosuria and osmotic polyuria are caused by hyperglycemia, which exceeds the ability of the kidneys to reabsorb glucose in the early stages of diabetes. First, the bladder adjusts, which increases the frequency of urination. Simultaneously, hyperglycemia induces increased oxidative phosphorylation in the bladder, as it does in all insulin-independent organs, leading to a considerable amount of oxidative stress. Excess reactive oxygen species, or free radicals, are produced when antioxidant defenses are not maintained. This imbalance leads to oxidative stress, which damages proteins, lipids, and DNA, among other parts of the cell [15].

DOI: http://dx.doi.org/10.5772/intechopen.1006899

The urothelium is composed of three distinct cellular strata: basal, intermediate, and apical/superficial. The highly differentiated cells of the superficial layer, also referred to as umbrella cells, serve as an essential barrier that obstructs the passage of toxins, ions, and water between urine and blood while also shielding the underlying excitable tissues from disturbance by urine constituents. The urothelium expresses a variety of receptors and produces signaling molecules, including nitric oxide (NO), ATP, and acetylcholine (ACh). The interaction between the urothelium and the underlying afferent innervation is hypothesized to be crucial in reflex responses to bladder filling and distension. Phenotypic alterations in the urothelium under pathological conditions can lead to diabetic bladder dysfunction [16]. Diabetic neuropathy is linked to either reduced nerve growth factor synthesis in the bladder or impaired nerve growth factor transport to the lumbosacral dorsal root ganglia. As diabetes progresses, chronic diabetic bladder dysfunction shows further symptoms of nonsensitivity and further failure of the bladder that results in overflow in voiding and high postvoid residual (PVR) volumes [15].

4.2 Effect of diabetes mellitus on an overactive/underactive bladder

4.2.1 Overactive bladder

Urinary frequency and nocturia are common symptoms of an overactive bladder, which is caused by involuntary contractions of the detrusor during the filling phase of the micturition cycle. It can occur with or without incontinence. Systemic inflammation, diabetes angiopathy, and neuropathy are the reasons for overactive bladder development in diabetic patients. These conditions all result in persistent ischemia of the bladder and central nervous system [17].

When the heightened glucose-filtered load from hyperglycemia surpasses the kidney's reabsorption capability (renal threshold), it causes osmotic diuresis, which increases urine production, leading to an overactive bladder [16].

4.2.2 Underactive bladder

An underactive bladder is unable to produce an efficient voiding contraction strong enough to empty the bladder, thereby resulting in lower urinary tract paralysis symptoms. The main cause of an Underactive Bladder is Detrusor Underactivity.

Diabetes may modify the contractile function of the detrusor muscle by affecting its myocytes and other components. As a result, even if the neural axis is still in position, the contractile force in the bladder is reduced. This could be the consequence of alterations to the detrusor muscle's excitation-contraction-coupling mechanisms, modifications to the ion storage and exchange system, or adjustments to the calcium storage and energy production systems [18].

5. Impact of diabetes mellitus on genital infections

A key issue for diabetes patients is that they have a highly weakened immune system, which makes it difficult for them to fight invading germs and increases their susceptibility to infections. *Candida albicans*, which is a yeast infection, is the most common cause of *Vulvovaginal candidiasis* (VVC) in women with diabetes [6]. Diabetes facilitates the attachment of yeast and other pathogens to skin cells and mucous glands. This can be the result of the presence of additional carbohydrates, which enables harmful yeast colonization. When diabetes is present, the body secretes more perspiration, mucus, and urine. Yeasts are nourished by sugars and thus thrive more in diabetic patients than in normal people. Additionally, increased amounts of glycogen, which is a polysaccharide that the body uses to store glucose, are also observed in diabetic patients. The accumulation of glycogen, especially in the vaginal region, may increase the acidity, which is a thriving condition for yeast infections. In individuals with compromised immune function due to conditions such as diabetes, yeast infection can become invasive if the infection is left untreated. It can travel through the circulation and affect other areas of the body, perhaps resulting in death.

Yeast infection-causing fungi are a common component of the vast array of microorganisms living inside our bodies. This fungus does not infect people unless it develops too much. There are also some diabetic drugs that can trigger the overgrowth of yeast in the genital tract, such as Invokana (canaglifozin) and Jardiance (empaglifozin) [19].

5.1 Role of hyperglycemia in promoting genital infections

The immune system modifications caused by hyperglycemia appear to be linked to mechanisms such as decreased inflammatory cytokine release, impaired T-cell and neutrophil activity, and decreased humoral immunity. This in turn causes the tissues to be more vulnerable to subsequent illness and infection. Inflammation that follows hyperglycemia is the primary cause of micro- and macroangiopathies in the circulatory system. They also promote fatty liver disease, increased intestinal permeability, and dysbiosis of the gut flora. Individuals with compromised immune systems and metabolic disorders are more vulnerable to many harmful substances [20].

6. Effect of diabetes mellitus on sexual dysfunction

6.1 Erectile dysfunction in men

The continuous inability to obtain or sustain a penile erection for successful sexual activity is known as erectile dysfunction.

Individuals with diabetes are at greater risk of sexual dysfunction, as long-term exposure to high blood sugar levels can harm neurons and blood vessels, including those that supply the male genital organ. A diabetic person suffering from erectile dysfunction may experience some loss of sensation as a result of this, limiting the blood flow to the genital organs and thereby leading to issues with arousal.

Elevated advanced glycation end-products and increased oxygen-free radical levels, decreased nitric oxide (NO) synthesis, increased endothelin B receptor binding sites, and ultrastructural alterations, upregulation of the RhoA/Rho-kinase pathway, NO-dependent selective nitrergic nerve degeneration, and impaired cyclic guanosine monophosphate-dependent kinase-1 are some of the hypothesized mechanisms of erectile dysfunction in diabetic patients [21].

6.2 Sexual dysfunction in women

In women with diabetes, the pathophysiology of female sexual dysfunction is intricate and multifaceted and involves both psychological and physiological factors [6].

Women experiencing sexual dysfunction may experience dyspareunia, poor lubrication, difficulty achieving an orgasm, and diminished libido [22].

Patients with diabetes mellitus can potentially have early signs of sexual dysfunction. Research suggests that silent coronary artery disease may manifest as male erectile dysfunction in its early stages. Therefore, it is speculated that in females, sexual dysfunction may be a precursor to coronary artery disease. Pathologically, hyperglycemia, vasculopathy, and neuropathy caused by type 2 diabetes mellitus result in female sexual dysfunction. Hyperglycemia causes membranes, especially vaginal tissues, to become less hydrated. This results in a decrease in lubrication and the development of dyspareunia with infections. Endothelial dysfunction arises from vascular changes caused by microangiopathy and atherosclerosis. At the very least of all, diabetic neuropathy modifies how people typically perceive and react to sexual stimuli [23].

6.3 Underlying biochemical processes contributing to sexual dysfunction in men and women

In some diabetic patients, apoptosis caused by the loss of BCT-2 expression in smooth muscle and increased connective tissue synthesis due to TGF beta decreases cavernosal tissue compliance by reducing or interfering with gap junctions and K channels in cavernosal smooth muscle, which are essential for coordinated cavernosal tissue relaxation in men.

Moreover, it is generally acknowledged that in the sympathetic nervous system, noradrenergic/noncholinergic neurotransmitters (NANCs), such as vasoactive intestinal polypeptide (VIP) and nitric oxide (NO), play major roles in sexual desire. Due to their basic involvement in the relaxation of the smooth muscles of vaginal tissues and subsequent increase in blood flow, these factors are responsible for controlling sexual function in females with diabetes.

Diabetes mellitus can cause a female genital organ to change both structurally and functionally. This can hinder the ability of genital tissues to relax and eventually cause problems with sexual function. Sexual relations can become unpleasant due to reduced clitoris engorgement and vaginal lubrication caused by other vascular abnormalities, such as malfunction of endothelial cells and atherosclerotic damage. Another prominent factor that contributes significantly to the pathophysiology of sexual problems is diabetic neuropathy. This may affect the way that sexual cues are normally transduced, as well as the resulting sexual response. The typical amounts of hormones such as androgens, estrogens, and sex hormone-binding globulin are out of balance [24].

6.4 Effect of diabetes mellitus on the menstrual cycle

Menstruation is the period during which the body sheds its uterine lining through the vagina, and progesterone and estrogen levels decrease. The interval between the first day of one menstrual cycle and the first day of the subsequent cycle is known as the menstrual cycle. Each person has a peculiar menstrual cycle. The typical menstrual cycle lasts for approximately 28 days [25].

The increased volume of body fat that results from diabetes causes people to produce more hormones, which in turn causes insulin resistance. The pancreas then produces even more insulin as a result. Hormones that control menstruation may combine with elevated insulin levels to cause irregular or absent menstruation. Even under rare circumstances, anovulation, which is the absence of ovulation, may occur [26].

7. Conclusion

In conclusion, the relationships between the biochemical processes of diabetes and urinary and genital tract alterations are complex and multifactorial. Diabetes, which is a result of hyperglycemia, can cause harm and dysfunction to the blood vessels, nerves, and tissues in these regions. The ensuing changes can manifest as genital tract alterations such as erectile dysfunction, low libido, and an increased risk of infections, as well as urinary issues such as frequent urination, urinary tract infections, and incontinence. Additionally, these changes may be worsened by diabetes-related inflammation and hormone abnormalities. It is crucial to know and remember that many illnesses can be successfully treated and avoided with appropriate diabetes care, routine screenings, and prompt interventions to prevent complications. Further studies and a complete understanding of the underlying biochemical pathways are crucial to improve the quality of life for individuals with diabetes and the alterations to the genital and urinary tract that are linked with diabetes.

Conflict of interest

The authors declare no conflicts of interest.

Author details

Oluwafemi Adeleke Ojo[1*], Tenifayo Soyinka[1], Emmanuel Henry Ezenabor[1] and Adebola Busola Ojo[2,3]

1 Department of Biochemistry, Bowen University, Iwo, Nigeria

2 Department of Environmental Management and Toxicology, University of Ilesa, Ilesa, Nigeria

3 Department of Biochemistry, Westland University, Iwo, Nigeria

*Address all correspondence to: oluwafemiadeleke08@gmail.com

References

[1] Sapra A. Diabetes [Internet]. 2023. Available from: https://www.ncbi.nlm.nih.gov/books/NBK551501/

[2] World Health Organization: WHO. Diabetes [Internet]. 2019. Available from: https://www.who.int/health-topics/diabetes#tab=tab_1

[3] Sweeting A, Wong J, Murphy H, Ross GP. A clinical update on gestational diabetes mellitus. Endocrine Reviews. 2022;**43**(5):763-793

[4] Sanches JM, Zhao L, Salehi A, Wollheim CB, Kaldis P. Pathophysiology of type 2 diabetes and the impact of altered metabolic interorgan crosstalk. The FEBS Journal. 2021;**290**(3):620-648

[5] Lović D, Piperidou A, Zografou I, Grassos H, Pittaras A, Manolis A. The growing epidemic of diabetes mellitus. Current Vascular Pharmacology. 2020;**18**(2):104-109

[6] Barbagallo F, Mongioì LM, Cannarella R, La Vignera S, Condorelli RA, Calogero AE. Sexual dysfunction in diabetic women: An update on current knowledge. Diabetology. 2020;**1**(1):11-21

[7] Boland BB, Rhodes CJ, Grimsby J. The dynamic plasticity of insulin production in β-cells. Molecular Metabolism. 2017;**6**(9):958-973

[8] Yau M. Treatment of Diabetes Mellitus in Children and Adolescents [Internet]. 2021. Available from: https://www.ncbi.nlm.nih.gov/books/NBK279087/

[9] Zakerkish M, Jenabi M, Zaeemzadeh N, Hemmati AA, Neisi N. The effect of Iranian propolis on glucose metabolism, lipid profile, insulin resistance, renal function and inflammatory biomarkers in patients with type 2 diabetes mellitus: A randomized double-blind clinical trial. Scientific Reports. 2019;**9**(1):7289

[10] Hatting M, Tavares CD, Sharabi K, Rines AK, Puigserver P. Insulin regulation of gluconeogenesis. Annals of the New York Academy of Sciences. 2017;**1411**(1):21-35

[11] Alsahli M, Gerich JE. Renal glucose metabolism in normal physiological conditions and in diabetes. Diabetes Research and Clinical Practice. 2017;**133**:1-9

[12] Kelley DE, Mokáň M, Veneman TF. Impaired postprandial glucose utilization in non-insulin-dependent diabetes mellitus. Metabolism. 1994;**43**(12):1549-1557

[13] Chainy G, Sahoo DK. Hormones and oxidative stress: An overview. Free Radical Research. 2019;**54**(1):1-26

[14] Jia Y, Liu Y, Feng L, Sun S, Sun G. Role of glucagon and its receptor in the pathogenesis of diabetes. Frontiers in Endocrinology. 2022;**13**:928016

[15] Inouye BM, Hughes FM, Jin H, Lütolf R, Potnis KC, Routh JC, et al. Diabetic bladder dysfunction is associated with bladder inflammation triggered through hyperglycemia, not polyuria. Research and Reports in Urology. 2018;**10**:219-225

[16] Hanna-Mitchell AT, Ruiz GW, Daneshgari F, Liu G, Apodaca G, Birder LA. Impact of diabetes mellitus on bladder uroepithelial cells. American Journal of Physiology-Regulatory Integrative and Comparative Physiology. 2013;**304**(2):84-93

[17] Zhu Y, Zhu Z, Chen J. Risk factors associated with the progression of overactive bladder among patients with type 2 diabetes. International Journal of Clinical Practice. 2019;**73**(11):e13395

[18] Aldamanhori R, Osman NI, Chapple CR. Underactive bladder: Pathophysiology and clinical significance. Asian Journal of Urology. 2018;**5**(1):17-21

[19] Wexler A. Diabetes and Yeast Infections (Candidiasis) [Internet]. 2023. Available from: https://www.medicalnewstoday.com/articles/317824

[20] Chávez-Reyes J, Escárcega-González CE, Chavira-Suárez E, León-Buitimea A, Vázquez-León P, Morones-Ramírez JR, et al. Susceptibility for some infectious diseases in patients with diabetes: The key role of glycemia. Frontiers in Public Health. 2021;**9**:559595

[21] Jumani D, Patil O. Erectile dysfunction in diabetes mellitus: A review. Journal of Diabetology: Official Journal of Diabetes in Asia Study Group. 2020;**11**(1):1

[22] Buskoven MEH, Kjørholt EKH, Strandberg RB, Søfteland E, Haugstvedt A. Sexual dysfunction in women with type 1 diabetes in Norway: A qualitative study of women's experiences. Diabetic Medicine. 2022;**39**(7):e14856

[23] Derosa G, Romano D, D'Angelo A, Maffioli P. Female sexual dysfunction in subjects with type 2 diabetes mellitus. Sexuality and Disability. 2023;**41**(2):221-233

[24] Singh R, Singh S, Jeyabalan G, Ali A, Semwal A. Medicinal plants used to treat sexual dysfunction: A review. International Journal of Recent Advances in Pharmaceutical Research. 2013;**3**:29-35

[25] Sissons B. How Does Diabetes Affect the Menstrual Cycle? [Internet]. 2021. Available from: https://www.medicalnewstoday.com/articles/does-diabetes-affect-period#the-menstrual-cycle

[26] Chisholm A. 5 Things Women Need to Know about Diabetes and their Period. Verywell Health [Internet]. 2023. Available from: https://www.verywellhealth.com/diabetes-and-womens-menstrual-cycles-4067212

Section 4

Innovations and Future

Chapter 8

Application of Data Science in Management of Type 1 Diabetes

Wenjing Meng, Jun Qin, Tixiao Wang and Ruxing Zhao

Abstract

Data science has now significantly penetrated the realm of Type 1 diabetes (T1D) management, offering invaluable assistance to healthcare providers in forecasting, monitoring, and treating the disease. Leveraging computer technology, Data science enables real-time monitoring or even predication of patients' blood sugar levels as well as complication development. By medical big data analytics involving patients' blood sugar, dietary habits, exercise patterns, and other relevant information, it contributes to personalized follow-up plans that are tailored to each patient's unique circumstances. Utilizing artificial intelligence (AI) algorithms, it also provides health management services, including health education and lifestyle guidance, to help patients better manage their diabetes and improve their quality of life. The AI-based individualized insulin-glucose precision regulation and response system (artificial pancreas) also provide precision insulin dosages in real time according to the real-time changes in glycemic levels and other physiological indicators, to maintain stable glycemic control. Moreover, integrated clinical and biological multi-omics data and application of machine learning (ML) grant researchers the capability to explore the genetic foundations, molecular pathways, and prospective therapeutic targets of T1DM with greater depth and precision. With continued technological advancements and deeper applications, Data science is expected to play an even greater role in the future.

Keywords: Data science, artificial intelligence, type 1 diabetes mellitus, machine learning, multi-omics, continuous subcutaneous insulin infusion, continuous glucose monitoring

1. Introduction

The management of Type 1 diabetes mellitus (T1DM) in clinical practice has historically been based on early epidemiological data and models depicting the natural progression of the disease. This methodology typically involves the periodic screening and follow-up of high-risk individuals and patients, often without a nuanced understanding of the precise timing and likelihood of beta-cell dysfunction, the onset of diabetes, and the subsequent development or worsening of complications. Moreover, traditional treatment approaches are devoid of personalized and precise directives for screening and follow-up schedules, as well as the absence of intelligent alert systems. Consequently, this results in a low percentage of patients actively engaging in monitoring and medical teams conducting proactive follow-ups. It also leads to the inefficient allocation of healthcare resources due to an excess of clinical interventions. These issues significantly compromise the ability to effectively regulate blood glucose levels in diabetic patients and the efficacy of preventive and therapeutic measures for complications, ultimately deteriorating patient outcomes and escalating the costs associated with managing these complications (**Figure 1**).

The emergence of the big data era in biomedicine has captured global interest, owing to the immense intrinsic value of its data. Programs, such as the Precision Medicine Initiative in the United States and the Healthy China 2030 strategy, have all placed a high priority on the vigorous advancement of bioinformatics and big data technology. Complex diseases like T1DM are characterized by multifaceted biological processes, encompassing genetic polymorphisms, environmental factor interactions (including viruses, medications, etc.), and intricate multi-level dynamics within the immune and metabolic systems, as well as in the epigenetic and metabolic profiles of organs. Clinically, the holistic management of T1DM is becoming increasingly sophisticated with the integration of a wide array of medical data, including blood glucose monitoring, insulin regimens, physical activity levels, dietary patterns, medical imaging, and clinical laboratory findings. Precision medicine seeks to leverage the analysis of large datasets to delineate the multifaceted progression of diseases across various biological informatics levels, revealing novel diagnostic, therapeutic targets, and biomarkers, thereby enhancing the precision and effectiveness of diagnoses, treatments as well as individualized management.

To tackle the complex nature of biomedical health data, characterized by its multi-source, heterogeneous, dynamic, and vast volumes, the creation of advanced, high-performance analytical models and methodologies is crucial for propelling the field of biomedical big data technology. This progress is indispensable for global health strategies, with bioinformatics playing a pivotal role in the efficient interpretation of high-dimensional biomedical datasets. Artificial intelligence (AI), including machine learning (ML), within the realm of computer science and technology, has paved the way for the closest approaches. Artificial intelligence has now significantly penetrated the realm of diabetes management, offering invaluable assistance to healthcare providers in forecasting, diagnosing, and treating the disease. It also plays a vital role in identifying potential complications and supports in glucose-level regulation. This innovative technology has the capacity to elevate the standards of healthcare delivery, promoting a more efficient and effective medical assessment process within the healthcare system. In the sphere of diabetes diagnostics, U.S. researchers have highlighted the promise of advanced high-dimensional machine learning techniques for predicting the incidence of Type 2 diabetes mellitus (T2DM). Through the application of the random forest algorithm, they integrated a comprehensive array of 93 variables, encompassing anthropometric indices, blood biomarkers, medical backgrounds, and echocardiographic findings. This integration facilitated the accurate anticipation of diabetes susceptibility among African Americans, as evidenced by an 8-year follow-up from the Jackson Heart Study. The fusion of professional knowledge, clinical acumen, and sophisticated machine learning methodologies has culminated in an efficacious risk assessment paradigm for diabetes. By inputting personal details, such as age, stature, body mass, and familial history, individuals can gauge their probability

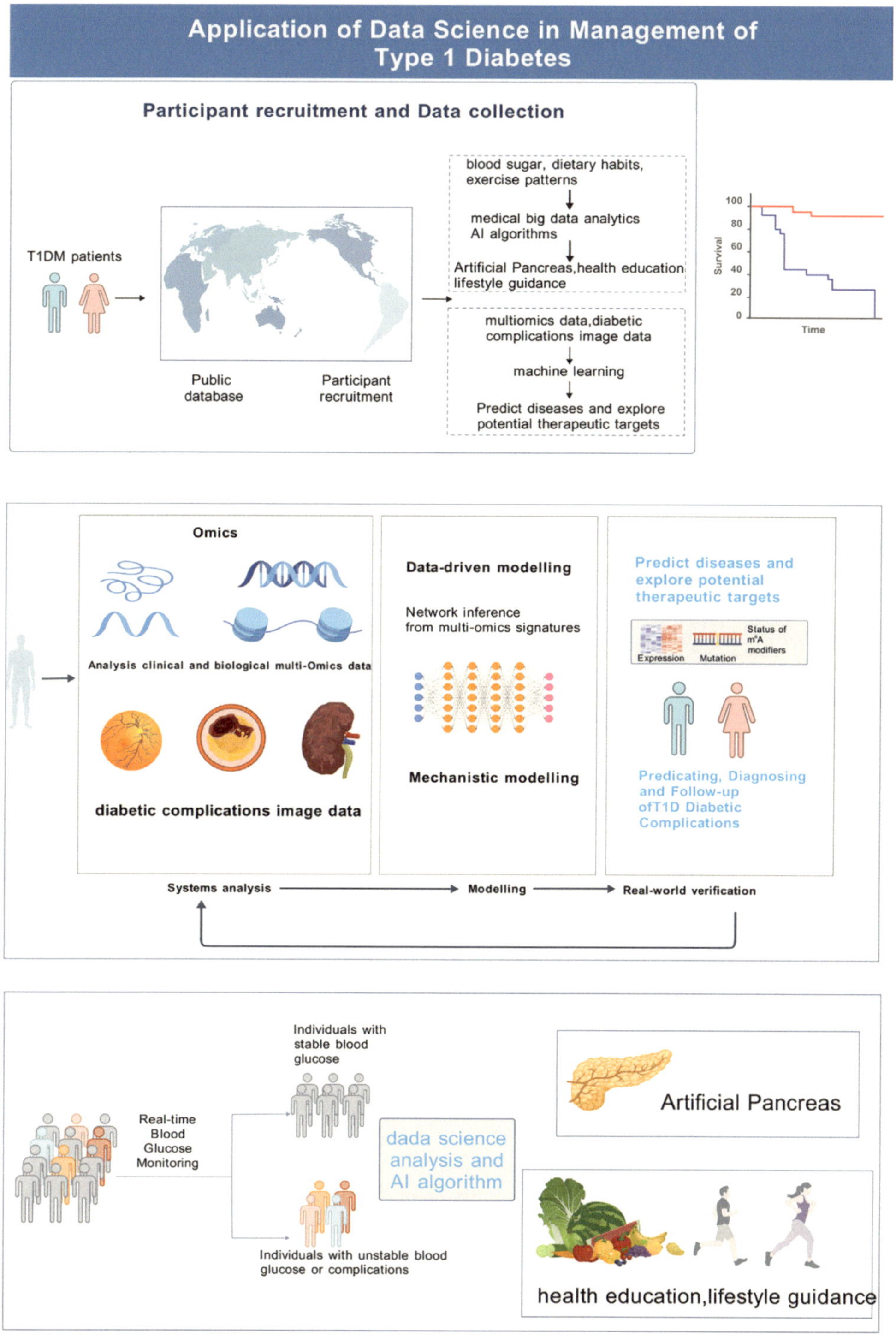

Figure 1.
Application of Data Science in management of Type 1 diabetes [1].

of diabetes onset within a 3-year horizon, thereby enabling tailored interventions and therapeutic strategies. The onset and progression of T1DM embody a seamless spectrum of dynamic physiological alterations, distinguished by unique cellular and molecular pathways at different phases. Cellular and molecular changes within each stage can profoundly affect the trajectory of subsequent disease progression. Nevertheless, the precise cellular molecules and signaling cascades that are pivotal during each disease phase—ranging from susceptibility, to immune activation in the presence of normal blood glucose levels, through early decompensation, to early and late-stage complications—remain poorly understood. This includes their influence on pancreatic beta-cell functionality, the distinct mechanisms of targeted organ damage within the context of hyperglycemia-induced harm, and the governance of these signaling elements in shaping the pathophysiologic conditions and disease trajectory at each diabetes stage, which are areas that merit further exploration. T1DM, in contrast to T2DM, is characterized by a lower incidence and prevalence, with a tendency to manifest at a younger age. It is governed by a multifaceted array of etiological and contributory elements, which complicates the collection of critical biological data, such as immune cell dynamics and antibody profiles. This complexity presents significant challenges in the realms of disease prediction and comprehensive management. Acknowledging the inadequacy of a reductionist, linear approach in diabetes research, an increasing contingent of investigators advocates for an integrative strategy. Modern T1DM research demands not only the utilization of conventional molecular and cellular biology techniques but also the incorporation of systems biology theories and methodologies from fields like genomics, proteomics, and metabolomics. This holistic approach aims to capture the intricacies and dynamic interplay of factors underlying T1DM, facilitating a deeper understanding of the disease.

However, at the global scale, the application of systems biology methodologies in T1DM research is still in its infancy. Landmark endeavors include the "Diabetes Genome Anatomy Project" initiated by American scholars in 2002 and the "Biological Atlas of Insulin Resistance" undertaken by British counterparts in 2003, both aligned with the systems biology paradigm. It is crucial to examine the network properties inherent in the pathogenesis and progression of T1DM through the lens of molecular networks, particularly by exploring functional genomics, gene regulatory networks, proteomics, and metabolomics in the context of diabetes.

In this chapter, we try to introduce and discuss the current progresses as well as future vista in the application of Data science in integrated management of T1D.

2. From risk stratifying to prediction of clinical onset of T1D by multi-omics data

T1DM is a chronic disease caused by progressive autoimmune destruction of the pancreatic β cells, leading to lifelong insulin dependence. The disorder has a genetic predisposition (stage 0) and can be identified in early presymptomatic stages such as stage 1, which represents individuals who have developed pancreatic autoimmunity with normoglycemia, and stage 2, which includes individuals who have progressed at a variable rate toward dysglycemia but remain asymptomatic or undiagnosed. Individuals who have become clinically symptomatic are considered stage 3. Recent and future progresses in available immunotherapies to delay or even block T1DM progression highlight the importance of identifying individuals at risk who might benefit from emerging treatments.

Although the etiology of the disease is still unknown, it is assumed that the autoimmune process is triggered by complex interactions between several genetic loci (nearly 60 loci described so far) and environmental factors. Prospective longitudinal studies of individuals at increased genetic risk have significantly advanced the understanding of the natural history of T1DM and characterized stages of disease progression. Identification of people at risk is increasingly relevant due to recent success in delaying clinical disease in presymptomatic individuals using immunotherapy.

Clinically, continuous glucose monitoring (CGM) is proved to be feasible and well tolerated in very young children at risk of T1DM since early dysglycemia is detectable using CGM in very young children at risk of T1DM. More importantly, omics technologies have significantly enhanced our understanding of the complex pathogenic mechanisms underlying T1DM. The latest breakthroughs in high-throughput omics, including genomics, transcriptomics, metabolomics, and proteomics, have granted researchers the capability to explore the genetic foundations, molecular pathways, and prospective therapeutic targets of T1DM with greater depth and precision.

Genomic research in T1DM is predominantly directed toward several pivotal domains. Genetic risk assessment leverages the-depth insights from genomic research to ascertain the hereditary susceptibility to T1DM by identifying and tracing the specific genetic alleles associated with the pathology. Empirical analysis of genetic variants has elucidated the pivotal role of select rare and low-frequency variants in conferring susceptibility to T1DM. Research has underscored that these variants often manifest a considerable effect size [2]. This discovery is instrumental in decoding the complex genetic framework of T1DM, holding the promise of novel therapeutic interventions. Furthermore, the exploration of the Cd101 gene within the non-obese diabetic (NOD) mouse model has pinpointed its critical role in the pathogenesis of T1DM [3]. Advances in genome-wide research have delineated the intricate pathogenic processes underlying T1DM. Associations between genetic variants and T1DM manifest diverse impacts across various age cohorts, with these variants located in proximity to genes pivotal for immune function and pancreatic β-cell physiology [4]. The studies led by Syreeni and associates have contributed significantly to the field through a comprehensive genome-wide meta-analysis, identifying specific genetic loci correlated with the timing of T1DM diagnosis. Their findings offer fresh insights into the role of these genes in both immune responses and the development of T1DM pathogenesis [5]. Genomic research delves into the complex interplay between genetic susceptibilities and environmental factors in the development of T1DM. Environmental factors, including aberrant intestinal microbiota, increased intestinal permeability, and altered mucosal immune responsiveness, interact with genetic predisposition to create a "perfect storm" for T1DM development [6]. Epigenetic modifications, such as DNA methylation and histone modifications, further modulate gene expression in T1DM [7]. The interplay between genetic background and environmental exposures throughout an individual's lifetime, including potential epigenetic inheritance, contributes to the complex etiology of diabetes [8]. The utilization of genomics in T1DM not only enhances the precision of early diagnosis and risk evaluation but also clarifies complex genetic-environmental interplays. This advancement provides a robust scientific basis for the formulation of individualized therapeutic regimens and proactive preventive interventions.

Transcriptomic and proteomic analyses are instrumental in probing T1DM, delineating the underlying molecular cascades and pinpointing prospective therapeutic targets. The Genetic Risk Score (GRS), when considered alongside specific islet autoantibody titers including insulinoma-2-associated autoantibodies (IA-2A), zinc transporter 8 autoantibodies (ZnT8A), and glutamic acid decarboxylase autoantibodies (GADA), emerges as a potent prognostic tool for evaluating the residual β-cell functionality in patients with T1DM. A composite biomarker model that integrates these indicators outperforms traditional predictors such as disease duration, age at onset, and GRS alone in forecasting the presence of C-peptide. This insight highlights the primacy of transcriptomic data in delineating disease trajectory and in maintaining β-cell integrity [9]. Additionally, the examination of plasma and immunoglobulin G (IgG) N-glycosylation profiles in patients recently diagnosed with T1DM has elucidated significant alterations in glycosylation structures linked to the disease's onset. These changes include an elevation in high-mannose and biantennary N-acetylglucosamine (GlcNAc) formations, coupled with a reduction in monogalactosylation. Research implies that these distinctive N-glycosylation patterns could serve as the basis for generating predictive models for T1DM, thereby refining the precision of risk assessment for this condition [10]. Proteomic investigations have delineated specific biomarkers and therapeutic candidates for T1DM by meticulously analyzing the proteomic expression landscapes. Metabolomic and proteomic approaches possess the robustness to identify and characterize metabolic substrates and protein biomarkers pertinent to T1DM. These encompass critical molecules, such as glucose, fructose, amino acids, and lipids, which demonstrate marked changes in individuals afflicted with T1DM. These distinctive biomarkers are instrumental in facilitating early detection and effective management of the condition [11]. High-resolution molecular phenotyping methodologies are instrumental in delineating the intricate associations between genetic variants and clinical phenotypes, shedding light on the underlying molecular pathways in T1DM. This research implies that proteomic information can be effectively leveraged to enhance the development of innovative therapeutic approaches and facilitate the advancement of disease surveillance tools [12]. Transcriptomics and proteomics play a pivotal role in the investigation of T1DM, elucidating the molecular mechanisms underlying the disease, identifying biomarkers, and furnishing a rationale for personalized therapeutic approaches. The comprehensive exploration of T-cell involvement in T1DM underscores the pivotal role of T-cell-related biomarkers in disease surveillance and therapeutic evaluation. These biomarkers are instrumental in advancing both the monitoring and management of T1DM. T-cell receptors (TCRs) function as identifiers of antigen specificity and, with the advent of advanced sequencing and computational analysis methods, have emerged as promising candidates for next-generation, non-cell-based biomarkers of T-cell responses. These biomarkers can act as surrogate markers for the existence of antigen-specific T cells. Studies suggest that TCR lineages and clonotypes demonstrate specificities in T1DM. Through the integration of comprehensive TCR datasets from T1DM patients and healthy individuals, coupled with sophisticated big data analytics, TCRs show potential as powerful indicators for the detection of T1DM [13]. Research indicates that calcium-independent phospholipase A2β (iPLA2β) is upregulated within the diabetic environment, and modulating its activity effectively reduces β-cell apoptosis. It has been observed that T cells with decreased iPLA2β expression can delay the onset of T1DM, improve glucose tolerance, and reduce the synthesis of pro-inflammatory lipids in an experiment of employing T-cell adoptive transfer strategy. These data imply that iPLA2β-derived pro-inflammatory lipids in CD4 T cells are critical factors in the pathogenesis of T1DM and may represent a promising therapeutic target [14]. Furthermore, mass cytometry has delineated distinct subsets of effector memory T regulatory cells and natural killer cells in individuals at elevated risk for T1DM. These cellular subsets are significantly increased in the high-risk population, indicating their promise as predictive biomarkers for the emergence of T1DM. This discovery deepens our comprehension of the participation of T cells in T1DM pathogenesis and identifies innovative targets for premature intervention strategies [15]. Research posits a pivotal role for the interplay between T and B cells in the etiology of T1DM. Notably, while signaling lymphocytic activation molecule-associated protein (SAP) is crucial in select autoimmune pathways, Tfh cells have been shown to function efficiently independent of SAP within the T1D context. This discovery implies that the pathogenicity of Tfh cells in T1DM is distinct from the traditional germinal center response, thereby presenting a novel insight into the immune dynamics of T1DM [16]. In conclusion, the exploration and utilization of T-cell-related biomarkers exhibit immense promise within the sphere of T1DM research. In-depth examination of T-cell receptor (TCR) diversity, iPLA2β expression, the role of regulatory T cells, and the interplay between T and B cells can significantly deepen our insight into the immune pathways that drive T1DM pathogenesis. Such insights are poised to expedite the progress toward more precise diagnostic strategies and potent therapeutic interventions for this condition.

Omics data integration plays a pivotal role in contemporary biomedical research, yet it confronts numerous complex challenges. These arise from the multifaceted nature of omics data, including genomics, transcriptomics, proteomics, and metabolomics, which exhibit significant heterogeneity in data formats, nomenclature, and spatiotemporal resolutions. During the preprocessing stage of machine learning, data integration is particularly sensitive to issues of quality and bias, striving to ensure that the integrated data meet the demands of analysis and model training [17]. Beyond a technical challenge, data integration also encompasses extensive collaborative efforts across social and organizational levels. Researchers from diverse disciplines and regions must achieve coordination in data collection, generation, and analysis to bridge discrepancies in hypotheses, methodologies, practices, and priorities [18]. When handling sensitive healthcare data, considerations of privacy and security become especially critical. In the face of numerous challenges associated with integrating omics data, the establishment of standards, technological advancements, and collaborative efforts across disciplines are poised to enhance the efficiency and integrity of future data integration endeavors. This progress is anticipated to significantly bolster advancements in biomedical research.

3. Real-time blood glucose monitoring and alerting by harnessing internet of things (IoT) and data science

Keeping blood glucose in the recommended range is central to the management for T1DM. This includes actively tracking blood glucose (BG) levels and managing physical activity, diet, insulin intake, and so on. For optimizing insulin therapy and glycemic control, close self-monitoring of blood glucose is essential. Continuous glucose monitoring (CGM) works by implanting sensors under the skin of the patient, which continuously monitors the glucose concentration in interstitial fluid and transmits the data to portable readers or smartphones, etc. Real-time blood glucose monitoring and alerting, enabled by the Internet of Things (IoT) and Data Science, is a rapidly evolving field that holds significant promise for improving the management of diabetes and enhancing patient outcomes. This technology combines the connectivity of IoT devices with the analytical power of Data Science to provide continuous, accurate, and personalized monitoring of blood glucose levels. This monitoring method can provide continuous and comprehensive glucose data, helping patients better manage their blood sugar control. The connectivity of IoT also enables seamless data transfer between the monitoring devices, patient smartphones, healthcare providers, and remote monitoring centers. Data Science plays a crucial role in processing and analyzing the vast amounts of data generated by IoT devices. Machine learning algorithms are used to identify patterns in glucose levels, predict hypoglycemic or hyperglycemic events, and personalize treatment recommendations. By analyzing historical data and patient behavior, Data Science can provide personalized insights into individual patients' glucose management needs. For example, algorithms can identify factors that contribute to blood sugar fluctuations, such as meal times, exercise, and medication intake.

At present, this CGM technology has been relatively mature and widely used in the clinical care of diabetic patients. Compared with traditional fingertip blood sugar monitoring, continuous glucose monitoring has the following advantages:

a. Provide more comprehensive glucose information: CGM can display the rising and falling trends of blood sugar, as well as the fluctuation range, which helps patients detect the risks of high and low blood sugar in time.

b. Reduce fingertip blood drawing: CGM can reduce the number of fingertip blood draws that patients need to do every day, reducing pain and inconvenience.

c. Improve blood sugar control quality: CGM can help patients better understand the impact of their diet, exercise, and medication on blood sugar, so they can adjust their lifestyle and improve blood sugar control quality. Tracking their glucose levels throughout the day, enabling earlier detection of hypoglycemic (low blood sugar) or hyperglycemic (high blood sugar) events.

d. Enhanced patient engagement: by providing continuous feedback, these systems encourage patients to take an active role in their health management. Data-driven insights also enable healthcare providers to tailor treatment plans to individual patients' needs.

e. Integration with other healthcare technologies: current developments have seen real-time blood glucose monitoring and alerting integrated with other IoT-enabled healthcare technologies, such as insulin pumps, to create closed-loop systems for automated glucose control.

Since the seminal study conducted by the Juvenile Diabetes Research Foundation (JDRF) in 2008, numerous randomized controlled trials have consistently demonstrated the superior efficacy of continuous glucose monitoring (CGM) over capillary finger sticks in terms of glycemic control [19, 20]. As a result, current guidelines now advocate for the integration of CGM as an essential component of standard care for individuals with Type 1 diabetes [21–23].

Two types of continuous glucose monitoring (CGM) are currently utilized in clinical practice: intermittently scanned CGM (isCGM) and real-time CGM (rtCGM). In contrast to first-generation isCGM, rtCGM, which features a transmitter that automatically transmits new glucose readings to a receiver, smartphone, or smartwatch every 1–5 minutes, is capable of emitting alarms for both high and low blood glucose levels. Furthermore, rtCGM alerts can be predictive as well as threshold-related, unlike the threshold-based alerts of second-generation isCGM. Observational and randomized controlled trials have demonstrated that rtCGM results in enhanced glycemic control and underscores the importance of alarms when making decisions about selecting CGM devices [24–26]. Clinical studies were conducted to investigate the potential additional benefits for adults with Type 1 diabetes when transitioning from first-generation isCGM without alerts to rtCGM with alert functionality [24, 27].

CGM is a comprehensive intervention that offers detailed information about glucose levels, including concentration, rate, and direction of change, historical trends, as well as alerts and alarms for potential or actual extreme fluctuations in glucose. Hybrid closed-loop systems are increasingly utilized by both adults and children with Type 1 diabetes, with CGM serving as a critical component of these systems. CGM significantly benefits individuals with Type 1 diabetes. Nevertheless, persistent challenges related to accessibility and user experience impede its widespread adoption and effectiveness. Such challenges involve the device's bulkiness, practical implementation difficulties, and societal stigma. Furthermore, issues like alarm fatigue, disrupted sleep patterns, and handling extensive real-time glucose data add to the complexity of CGM usage. A more tailored approach to continuous glucose monitoring could amplify its advantages and ease the self-care requirements for users. Moreover, healthcare providers' subconscious biases concerning patients' socioeconomic status, educational background, age, ethnicity, and other demographic factors might influence their distribution of continuous glucose monitors [28].

Blood glucose prediction approaches can be broadly classified into three major categories: physiology-based, data-driven, and hybrid methods [29–31]. CGM and other point-of-care (POC) devices for self-monitoring and management purposes have facilitated the generation of automated and continuous personal data. This has created an opportunity to leverage more detailed datasets for enhancing the training of machine learning models. Data science and machine learning techniques have been employed to predict BG, including feed-forward neural networks [32], deep neural networks [33], Gaussian processes [34], support vector machines [35], genetic algorithms and programming [36], and self-organizing maps [37]; these methodologies utilize diverse groups of input parameters and training algorithms [38].

With advancements in Data science and in response to the therapeutic needs of Type 1 diabetes, the trajectory of CGM technology is aimed at achieving predictive modeling of blood glucose and dynamic modeling of blood glucose fluctuations. However, due to the complexity of blood glucose dynamics, it remains challenging to develop a universal model that can provide accurate predictions under free-living conditions and in all circumstances. Besides, ensuring the safe and secure handling of sensitive patient data is a critical challenge.

4. Application of data science in predicating, diagnosing, and follow-up of T1D's diabetic complications

The advent of computer-aided diagnostic tools and deep learning algorithms has also shown tremendous potential in the detection of diabetic complications. Artificial intelligence (AI) and big data are revolutionizing the detection, management, and treatment of diabetic retinopathy (DR) in patients with diabetes mellitus. AI-enabled systems using retinal images have been clinically adopted for high-throughput DR screening, offering potential for holistic diabetes care and risk prognostication of cardiovascular complications [39]. These AI tools provide low-cost, effective solutions for early and accurate diagnosis, supporting specialists and treatment selection [40]. AI applications extend to monitoring DR progression, predicting treatment outcomes, and risk stratification for vision-threatening DR and diabetic macular edema [41]. Furthermore, AI and telehealth can improve access, financial sustainability, and coverage of DR screening programs, facilitating the integration of community, primary, and specialist eye care services [42]. As diabetes prevalence continues to rise globally, AI-assisted retinal image analysis has the potential to become a central tool in modern personalized medicine for diabetic patients. The sophisticated deep learning systems have demonstrated high levels of sensitivity and specificity in the identification of diabetic retinopathy and associated ocular pathologies. Their adaptability across diverse patient cohorts and varying clinical scenarios is particularly noteworthy. Gulshan and associates developed a pioneering deep learning-based screening software, EyePACS-1, which achieved an impressive diagnostic performance for diabetic retinopathy with a sensitivity of 90.3%, a specificity of 98.1%, and an area under the receiver operating characteristic (ROC) curve of 0.99, using a reference standard of moderate to severe retinopathy or diabetic macular edema. In a similar vein, Gargeya's work brought to light a purely data-driven artificial intelligence grading algorithm for the screening of diabetic fundus pathology, which exhibited high dependability with a sensitivity of 94%, a specificity of 98%, and an area under the ROC curve of 0.97.

While not a substitute for definitive diagnosis, the artificial intelligence screening system for diabetic retinopathy offers valuable support to ophthalmologists, particularly in regions with scarce medical resources. It significantly contributes to the reduction of healthcare costs, minimizes uncertainty in clinical decision-making, and obviates subjective biases in expert assessments. Beyond retinopathy, confocal microscopy is increasingly being utilized for the diagnosis of diabetic neuropathy, and the imaging of lower limb lesions in diabetes is greatly enhanced by the application of image processing in lower limb vascular ultrasound. Intelligent computer-aided systems are poised to play a crucial role in the mass, rapid, and precise screening of these complications, thereby revolutionizing diagnostic capabilities in the field.

Deep learning approaches have showcased substantial prowess in the realm of large-scale image processing, particularly in the domain of medical imaging, where rapid advancements have been witnessed. Given the well-established diagnostic criteria for diabetic retinopathy and its comprehensive classification system, it is feasible to compile an extensive dataset. This has led to the intense focus of research on leveraging deep learning algorithms for the diagnosis of this condition. In 2016, Google successfully applied the Inception-v3 architecture, achieving impressive sensitivity rates of 90.3 and 87.0%, along with high specificity levels of 98.1 and 98.5% in two separate validation studies.

In the realm of diagnosing diabetic retinopathy, the predominant imaging techniques include color fundus photography (CFP), optical coherence tomography (OCT), and optical coherence tomography angiography (OCTA). The synthesis of these multi-modal imaging datasets has significantly augmented diagnostic precision, thanks to technological progress and the widespread access to such equipment. Nonetheless, this integration has concurrently multiplied the professional workload, highlighting the indispensable role of sophisticated, automated systems designed to facilitate multi-modal diagnostic assistance.

Recent studies have explored the application of artificial intelligence (AI) and machine learning (ML) in predicting and managing diabetic kidney disease (DKD) in Type 1 diabetes. AI-based models using electronic medical records have shown promise in predicting DKD progression with 71% accuracy [43] and an AUC of 0.74 [44]. These models incorporate various features, including time series data and natural language processing. A systematic review identified limited studies specifically focusing on ML for predicting microvascular complications in Type 1 diabetes, with common predictors including age, gender, diabetes duration, and HbA1C levels [45]. Popular ML algorithms used in these studies include random forest, support vector machines, and neural networks. Another review highlighted that AI frameworks often outperform conventional statistical methods in diagnosing and treating DKD, though limitations such as lack of external validation were noted [46].

Unfortunately, the existing contributions of Data science to the realm of T1DM diagnosis and treatment primarily center on identifying established diseases. Nonetheless, the creation of precise predictive models for diabetes and its related complications could markedly improve the recognition of high-risk groups, forecast the emergence of the disease, and potentially provide significant added value to the integrated management and tertiary prevention strategies for T1DM, despite the increased complexities involved.

5. Application of AI Technologies in Health Education and Individualized Healthcare Management of T1D

The deployment of artificial intelligence (AI) in the management of Type 1 Diabetes (T1D) is chiefly aimed at augmenting the effectiveness and ease of insulin treatment. It also involves the provision of tailored decision-making assistance to help patients attain optimal glycemic regulation.

For example, the development of a Health Education Support System leveraging virtual reality (VR) technology facilitates the creation of an authentic sensory environment through computational simulation. This allows participants to engage with virtual elements using human sensory-motor skills, such as head and eye movements, gestures, and other actions. Characterized by its immersive, interactive, and constructive experiences, VR effectively mirrors real-world processes. For those at the grassroots level suffering from chronic diseases, who typically possess lower levels of education and exhibit limited responsiveness to health education, VR emerges as a potent tool. By using VR equipment, these individuals can virtually experience scenarios including proper eating habits, physical exercises, and medication adherence, thereby swiftly absorbing correct lifestyle and pharmaceutical usage techniques. In the realm of diabetes education at the community level, VR can replicate dietary regimens, guiding patients on the appropriate balance of carbohydrates, fats, proteins, and fiber. Additionally, it can simulate physical activities, advising on the choice of aerobic and resistance exercises and managing intensity levels. The imitation of medication dosing can also instruct patients on the correct timing, dosage, and administration methods. This empowers patients to independently explore and practice within a dynamic, interactive, and virtual space, significantly enhancing their self-care abilities.

A sophisticated, mobile internet-based platform is used for the comprehensive management of chronic diseases, underpinned by big data-driven intelligence and precision.

Intelligent data collection enhances the procurement of inclusive, continuous, and multifaceted personal health information. This integration involves an array of smart medical devices, such as blood glucose meters, blood pressure monitors, smartwatches, and body composition scales, ensuring a holistic capture of health-related data. This comprehensive approach extends beyond hospital environments to external facilities like health clinics, pharmacies, and domestic settings. Such seamless data aggregation facilitates persistent health monitoring, enabling sophisticated health assessments, accurate health condition identification, and stratified patient care management.

We can employ sophisticated intelligence analytics to dissect patient visit patterns, physical examination results, and physician follow-up data, thereby crafting bespoke health profiles that quantify personal health metrics. Currently, by relying on large databases based on real-world studies, AI-based chronic disease diagnosis and treatment models can be built using convolutional neural networks, recurrent neural networks, and other deep learning algorithms. Based on individual disease subtypes and risk levels, the models can intelligently generate personalized health management plans and recommend diet, exercise, and insulin application, among other multi-dimensional health behavior intervention management solutions, to improve health levels. Through intelligent matching of diagnostic and treatment models, AI can recommend personalized and precise health management paths for patients and healthcare professionals. Through the application of advanced predictive analytical models, we are able to evaluate and project patient health statuses, deploying tiered management approaches. This integration of empirical disease assessment with comprehensive health records enables us to produce nuanced condition evaluations, providing trend analysis and forecasting the trajectory of disease advancement.

Sophisticated AI diagnostic models enable accurate matching and tailor-made precision healthcare pathway suggestions. Utilizing advanced deep learning techniques such as convolutional neural networks and recurrent neural networks, these systems establish AI-driven diagnostic frameworks specifically for chronic illnesses. They adaptively devise personalized health programs by considering unique disease profiling and diverse risk factors. These strategies provide customized interventions encompassing dietary, physical activity, and sleep regimens, thereby elevating the standards of holistic health management to an individualized, "thousand-persons-thousand-paths" approach.

Customized typing follow-up administration enhances the efficiency and automation of medical follow-ups for healthcare professionals. This system adapts to the diverse conditions among patient cohorts by creating bespoke follow-up protocols that vary in both frequency and detail. These protocols integrate critical information such as the timing and specifics of each follow-up. Through the implementation and documentation of patient progress and the analysis of their test results, the system alerts physicians to intervene, when necessary. Simultaneously, it independently adapts the follow-up pathway and schedules in response to changes in individual patient status and updates to their treatment history.

6. Development of artificial pancreas (AP) systems

Continuous glucose monitoring (CGM) systems, coupled with automated insulin delivery (AID) systems, have exhibited significant promise and therapeutic efficacy in the regulation and management of diabetes, offering a sophisticated approach to maintaining glycemic control, particularly for type 1 diabetes. AID systems, comprising a CGM, insulin pump, and control algorithm, have demonstrated improved glycemic outcomes and time in range [47]. These systems automate basal insulin delivery and some offer automatic correction boluses, reducing the burden on patients [48]. Multiple AID options are now commercially available, with more in development [49]. CGM technology has also evolved to integrate with connected insulin pens and virtual platforms, showing benefits in both Type 1 and Type 2 diabetes [50]. Future developments may incorporate additional hormones, activity levels, and artificial intelligence to further optimize diabetes management [48, 50]. As CGM accuracy improves and AID systems become more sophisticated, they hold promise for broadly achieving goal-level glycemic control while minimizing hypoglycemia risk [49, 50].

Artificial pancreas (AP) systems are closed-loop devices that aim to automate glucose control in Type 1 diabetes. These systems integrate continuous glucose sensors, insulin pumps, and control algorithms to mimic pancreatic function [51]. Clinical trials have demonstrated the feasibility and efficacy of AP systems in various settings, from supervised to free-living conditions [52]. Studies have shown improved glycemic outcomes, reduced hypoglycemia risk, and positive user acceptance across different age groups, including children, adolescents, adults, and pregnant women [53]. Additionally, closed-loop systems have significantly improved the well-being of patients suffering from a range of chronic illnesses. These advanced systems leverage intelligent and digitized management strategies to bolster patients' self-care abilities and enhance their overall quality of life. Moreover, they succeed in minimizing the occurrence of complications, providing a scalable model for effective chronic disease management. As of 2015, 18 closed-loop AP systems were in development, with some expected to become commercially available in the following years [54]. The approval of the first hybrid closed-loop system in 2016 marked a significant advancement in AP technology [53]. Rigorous research has confirmed the robust efficacy of these closed-loop algorithms across diverse scenarios, encompassing daily activities, pregnancy, and in different demographic segments. As technological progress continues apace, the potential applications for closed-loop systems have experienced a substantial broadening. The synergy between artificial intelligence and sophisticated decision-support mechanisms is poised to further augment the efficacy and user satisfaction of these systems. Ongoing and future research is expected to focus on dual-hormone regulation and the development of fully automated closed-loop systems that operate without the need for pre-meal alerts. These breakthroughs promise to markedly enhance the management of Type 1 diabetes, offering a new horizon of convenience and control for patients [55]. The closed-loop algorithm for artificial pancreas has emerged as a potent strategy in the efficient management of Type 1 diabetes, offering a spectrum of distinctive advantages. Nonetheless, it confronts several pivotal challenges that necessitate thorough resolution. These include issues of systemic reliability, patient acceptance, and long-term safety considerations. In reaction to these hurdles, an ongoing commitment to research, complemented by relentless technological progress, is aimed at surmounting these obstacles. The overarching objective is to refine the closed-loop system's efficacy, guaranteeing its optimized performance and superior therapeutic results for those suffering from Type 1 diabetes.

7. Discussion

From the stratification of risk to the prediction of clinical onset of T1D through multi-omics data analysis, the application of genomic technologies has significantly enhanced our profound comprehension of the intricate pathogenic mechanisms underlying T1DM. Leveraging the latest advancements in high-throughput omics, including genomics, transcriptomics, metabolomics, and proteomics, researchers are now able to explore the genetic backdrop, molecular pathways, and potential therapeutic targets for T1DM with greater refinement and precision. Integrating omics technologies with artificial intelligence is poised to significantly enhance research into Type 1 diabetes mellitus (T1DM) and improve its management. Omics data, rich in complex biological information, can be effectively processed and deeply analyzed by AI algorithms, revealing the underlying mechanisms of the disease and opening new paths for therapeutic development.

The real-time continuous glucose monitoring system affords a continuous and comprehensive dataset, enabling patients to manage their blood sugar levels with greater precision. Leveraging the interconnectedness of the Internet of Things, the system ensures seamless data transmission among monitoring devices, patients' smartphones, healthcare providers, and remote monitoring centers. Data science is indispensable in processing and analyzing the vast quantities of data generated by IoT devices, with machine learning algorithms employed to discern patterns in glucose-level fluctuations, predict hypoglycemic or hyperglycemic events, and accordingly offer personalized therapeutic recommendations.

Artificial intelligence-enabled retinal image analysis significantly enhances the efficiency of high-throughput screening for diabetic retinopathy, enabling cost-effective and expedient early diagnosis as well as accurate risk prediction. This technology not only monitors the progression of DR but also forecasts therapeutic outcomes and stratifies patient risks. Confocal microscopy serves as a valuable tool in diagnosing diabetic neuropathy, while advanced image processing techniques in lower limb ultrasound imaging refine lesion visualization. Computer-aided diagnostic systems are poised to revolutionize the mass screening of diabetic complications. Furthermore, AI and machine learning models, leveraging electronic medical records, exhibit promise in predicting the progression of DKD in Type 1 diabetes. The integration of AI with telemedicine has the potential to improve the accessibility, financial viability, and reach of screening initiatives for diabetic complications, thereby facilitating the convergence of community-based, primary, and specialized ophthalmic care services.

Supported by the intelligentization and precision enabled by big data, this comprehensive chronic disease management platform is anchored in the mobile internet. An educational health support system, developed through virtual reality technology, empowers patients to independently explore and practice rational dietary plans, appropriate exercise intensity, accurate medication timing, dosage, and administration in an interactive and virtual environment, significantly enhancing their self-care capabilities. Leveraging deep learning algorithms such as convolutional neural networks and recurrent neural networks, we can customize personal health records and smartly generate health management plans based on disease subtypes and risk levels, achieving personalized health interventions, assessing and predicting health status, and optimizing treatment pathways.

The artificial pancreas (AP) system, an advanced closed-loop apparatus, is designed to automate glycemic control in patients with Type 1 diabetes. It incorporates dynamic glucose sensors, insulin pumps, and sophisticated control algorithms to emulate the normal function of the pancreas. Rigorous research has demonstrated the efficacy of these closed-loop algorithms across diverse scenarios, including daily life, pregnancy, and varied demographic characteristics. With technological advancements, the potential applications of closed-loop systems have significantly expanded.

The integration of artificial intelligence with advanced decision-support systems heralds a further enhancement in system performance and user satisfaction. Current and future studies will focus on the development of dual-hormone regulation mechanisms and fully automated closed-loop systems without pre-meal alerts. These technological breakthroughs are poised to substantially improve the management of Type 1 diabetes, offering patients a more convenient and autonomous control solution.

Data science and artificial intelligence have demonstrated unparalleled advantages in the early diagnosis, precision treatment, and prediction of complications for Type 1 diabetes, harboring immense potential for development. Nonetheless, the realization of these benefits is accompanied by numerous challenges. In terms of disease prediction, the acquisition of data presents significant difficulties, and the generalization capability of models is limited. The pathogenesis of Type 1 diabetes is complex, involving genetic, environmental, and immunological factors, making it challenging to obtain comprehensive, high-quality data. Moreover, due to the variability in disease characteristics among different regions and populations, the stability of models across diverse datasets is insufficient. In the diagnostic realm, AI diagnostic models are susceptible to misdiagnosis and missed diagnoses, particularly in accurately identifying early or atypical cases of Type 1 diabetes. Furthermore, the interpretation of AI diagnostics is highly dependent on medical expertise, necessitating integration with professional judgments from physicians. During treatment, the development of personalized therapeutic regimens for patients with Type 1 diabetes is complex, and the assessment of treatment efficacy requires long-term tracking and multidimensional data analysis. AI may face limitations when handling these complex datasets. In predicting and treating complications of Type 1 diabetes, AI must manage substantial amounts of intricate data, and the variability in treatment needs for complications among different patients poses significant challenges in devising personalized therapeutic plans.

The application of Data science and artificial intelligence is not an ultimate objective. Our central tenet is to leverage the technological advantages of the big data era to enhance the efficiency and accuracy of diabetes diagnosis and treatment. Establishing a cross-regional, cross-institutional data sharing platform, amalgamating diverse data resources, optimizing data integrity and quality, and reinforcing data integration and sharing mechanisms. Employing advanced techniques such as multi-task learning and transfer learning to enhance model adaptability and stability across different datasets, thereby improving model generalization capabilities. Integrating multi-dimensional information, including clinical data, genomics, and metabolomics, to enhance the accuracy and reliability of artificial intelligence diagnosis. Creating a collaborative working model between doctors and artificial intelligence, where AI provides auxiliary diagnostic suggestions, and doctors make final decisions based on their professional knowledge and experience. Utilizing machine learning and deep learning techniques to develop algorithms capable of customizing personalized treatment plans according to individual patient characteristics. Establishing a long-term tracking and evaluation system for patients, collecting data during treatment to continuously refine therapeutic regimens. Constructing a knowledge graph encompassing various complications and related information to aid artificial intelligence in more accurately understanding and processing complication data. Strengthening interdisciplinary collaboration among endocrinology, cardiology, nephrology, and other departments to jointly research and develop intelligent diagnostic and treatment solutions for Type 1 diabetes complications.

Some research papers also highlight the critical role of Sirtuin 1 (Sirt 1), an anti-aging gene, in various chronic diseases. Sirt 1 is involved in appetite regulation, cell senescence, and apoptosis, with its suppression linked to insulin resistance, non-alcoholic fatty liver disease (NAFLD), and neurodegenerative diseases [56]. Nutritional interventions and calorie restriction early in life can maintain Sirt 1 and other anti-aging genes, potentially improving metabolic health [56]. Environmental factors, including unhealthy diets and bacterial lipopolysaccharides, can inactivate Sirt 1, leading to immune system alterations, NAFLD, and diabetes [57]. The interplay between Sirt 1 and nitric oxide is relevant to autoimmune diseases and multiple organ dysfunction syndrome (MODS) [57]. Sirt 1 is also crucial in diagnostic proteomics, serving as a biomarker for chronic disease progression and therapeutic drug efficacy, particularly in diabetes and neurodegenerative diseases [58].

8. Conclusions

In summary, the application of Data science in the management of T1D is becoming increasingly important. Undoubtedly, the progress of Data science will greatly facilitate both scientific research and clinical practice in T1DM. Of course, subsequent inquiry should also concentrate on the synthesis and data extrapolation from diabetes-related omics data, molecular interaction networks, and the kinetic signaling pathways. Such endeavors are likely to clarify the disease's network dynamics, disclose the underpinning mechanisms of T1DM onset and advancement, and yield a treasure trove of multi-omics insights. Another goal is to develop a seamless, cost-efficient open-service platform for conditional data, catering to both healthcare professionals and patients. Ultimately, these studies are expected to pave the way for more complex and advanced diagnostic and therapeutic support systems in clinical practice. It can be anticipated that in the near future, Data science such as AI is expected to help us build a seamless, cost-effective open-service platform for Type 1 diabetes patients and healthcare professionals to meet the needs of medical professionals and patients. This platform will completely change the traditional T1DM management method by shifting from a disease-focused model to an integrated model of real-time monitoring, adjustable interventions, and information technology-based infrastructure. These approaches will provide comprehensive and multifaceted care throughout the entire spectrum of T1DM. The plan will also cover tiered diagnostic and treatment strategies, alongside the dissemination of health-related knowledge.

Acknowledgements

In this context, we extend our profound gratitude to all the scholars whose works have been referenced in the present paper, as well as to the investigators in contiguous disciplines whose erudite contributions have bolstered the scholarly underpinnings of this research endeavor. Additionally, we convey our heartfelt appreciation for the comprehensive informational assets afforded by the library and the digital reading room.

This work was supported by the National Natural Science Foundation of China (82370853 and 82070868).

Conflict of interest

The authors declare no conflict of interest.

Author details

Wenjing Meng[1,2,3], Jun Qin[1,2,3], Tixiao Wang[1,2,3] and Ruxing Zhao[1,2,3]*

1 Department of Endocrinology and Metabolism, Qilu Hospital of Shandong University, China

2 Shandong Provincial Key Laboratory of Spatiotemporal Regulation and Precision Intervention in Endocrine and Metabolic Diseases, China

3 Shandong Provincial Engineering Research Center for Advanced Technologies in Prevention and Treatment of Chronic Metabolic Diseases, Jinan, China

*Address all correspondence to: ruxingzhao@mail.sdu.edu.cn

References

[1] Created with BioGDP.com

[2] Pang H, Xia Y, Luo S, Huang G, Li X, Xie Z, et al. Emerging roles of rare and low-frequency genetic variants in type 1 diabetes mellitus. Journal of Medical Genetics. 2021;**58**(5):289-296

[3] Mattner J, Mohammed JP, Fusakio ME, Giessler C, Hackstein C-P, Opoka R, et al. Genetic and functional data identifying Cd101 as a type 1 diabetes (T1D) susceptibility gene in nonobese diabetic (NOD) mice. PLoS Genetics. 2019;**15**(6):e1008178-e

[4] Inshaw JRJ, Cutler AJ, Crouch DJM, Wicker LS, Todd JA. Genetic variants predisposing most strongly to type 1 diabetes diagnosed under age 7 years lie near candidate genes that function in the immune system and in pancreatic β-cells. Diabetes Care. 2020;**43**(1.0):169-177

[5] Syreeni A, Sandholm N, Sidore C, Cucca F, Haukka J, Harjutsalo V, et al. Genome-wide search for genes affecting the age at diagnosis of type 1 diabetes. Journal of Internal Medicine. 2021;**289**(5):662-674

[6] Vaarala O, Atkinson MA, Neu J. The "perfect storm" for type 1 diabetes. Diabetes. 2008;**57**:2555-2562

[7] Stankov K, Benc D, Drašković D. Genetic and epigenetic factors in etiology of diabetes mellitus type 1. Pediatrics. 2013;**132**:1112-1122

[8] Tremblay J, Hamet P. Environmental and genetic contributions to diabetes. Metabolism: Clinical and Experimental. 2019;**100S**:153952

[9] Williams MD, Bacher R, Perry DJ, Grace CR, McGrail KM, Posgai AL, et al. Genetic composition and autoantibody titers model the probability of detecting C-peptide following type 1 diabetes diagnosis. The Journal of Maternal-Fetal & Neonatal Medicine: The Official Journal of the European Association of Perinatal Medicine, the Federation of Asia and Oceania Perinatal Societies, the International Society of Perinatal Obstetricians. 2021;**70**(4):932-943

[10] Najda R, Domagoj K, Simranjeet K, Vesna S, Ana C, Flemming P, et al. Children at onset of type 1 diabetes show altered N-glycosylation of plasma proteins and IgG. Diabetologia. 2022;**65**(8):1315-1327

[11] Arneth B, Arneth R, Shams M. Metabolomics of type 1 and type 2 diabetes. International Journal of Molecular Sciences. 2019;**20**(10):2467

[12] Franks PW, Pomares-Millan H. Next-generation epidemiology: The role of high-resolution molecular phenotyping in diabetes research. Diabetologia. 2020;**63**(12):2521-2532

[13] Nakayama M, Michels AW. Using the T cell receptor as a biomarker in type 1 diabetes. Frontiers in Immunology. 2021;**12**:777788

[14] White T, Chalfant C, Dilorenzo TP, Ramanadham S, Stephenson D. 74-OR: Adoptively transferred T lymphocytes with reduced Ipla2b expression delays type 1 diabetes development in NOD mice. Diabetes. 2022;**71**(Suppl. 1):74

[15] Barcenilla H, Åkerman L, Pihl M, Ludvigsson J, Casas R. Mass cytometry identifies distinct subsets of regulatory T cells and natural killer cells associated with high risk for type 1 diabetes. Frontiers in Immunology. 2019;**10**:982

[16] Bonami RH, Nyhoff LE, McNitt DH, Hulbert C, Felton JL, Kendall PL, et al. T–B lymphocyte interactions promote type 1 diabetes independently of SLAM-associated protein. The Journal of Immunology. 2020;**205**(12):3263-3276

[17] Nargesian F, Asudeh A, Jagadish H. Responsible data integration: Next-generation challenges. In: Proceedings ACM-Sigmod International Conference on Management of Data. Association for Computing Machinery (ACM); 2022

[18] Neang AB, Sutherland W, Beach MW, Lee CP. Data Integration as Coordination: The Articulation of Data Work in an Ocean Science Collaboration. New York, USA: Association for Computing Machinery; 2020. 1-25 p

[19] Maiorino MI, Signoriello S, Maio A, Chiodini P, Bellastella G, Scappaticcio L, et al. Effects of continuous glucose monitoring on metrics of glycemic control in diabetes: A systematic review with meta-analysis of randomized controlled trials. Diabetes Care. 2020;**43**(5):1146-1156

[20] Dicembrini I, Cosentino C, Monami M, Mannucci E, Pala L. Effects of real-time continuous glucose monitoring in type 1 diabetes: A meta-analysis of randomized controlled trials. Acta Diabetologica. 2021;**58**(4):401-410

[21] Holt RIG, DeVries JH, Hess-Fischl A, Hirsch IB, Kirkman MS, Klupa T, et al. The management of type 1 diabetes in adults. A consensus report by the American Diabetes Association (ADA) and the European Association for the Study of diabetes (EASD). Diabetologia. 2021;**64**(12):2609-2652

[22] National Institute for Health and Care Excellence. Type 1 diabetes in adults: Diagnosis and management. 2015. Available from: https://www.nice.org.uk/guidance/ng17/chapter/Recommendations#blood-glucosemanagement [Accessed: May 5, 2022]

[23] ElSayed NA, Aleppo G, Bannuru RR, Bruemmer D, Collins BS, Ekhlaspour L, et al. 7. Diabetes technology: Standards of care in diabetes-2024. Diabetes Care. 2023;**47**(Suppl. 1):S126-SS44

[24] Visser MM, Charleer S, Fieuws S, De Block C, Hilbrands R, Van Huffel L, et al. Comparing real-time and intermittently scanned continuous glucose monitoring in adults with type 1 diabetes (ALERTT1): A 6-month, prospective, multicentre, randomised controlled trial. Lancet. 2021;**397**(10291):2275-2283

[25] Reddy M, Jugnee N, El Laboudi A, Spanudakis E, Anantharaja S, Oliver N. A randomized controlled pilot study of continuous glucose monitoring and flash glucose monitoring in people with type 1 diabetes and impaired awareness of hypoglycaemia. Diabetic Medicine. 2018;**35**(4):483-490

[26] Seibold A. Comment on Hásková et al. real-time CGM is superior to flash glucose monitoring for glucose control in type 1 diabetes: The CORRIDA randomized controlled trial. Diabetes care 2020;43:2744-2750. Diabetes Care. 2021;**44**(4):e75-ee6

[27] Visser MM, Charleer S, Fieuws S, De Block C, Hilbrands R, Van Huffel L, et al. Effect of switching from intermittently scanned to real-time continuous glucose monitoring in adults with type 1 diabetes: 24-month results from the randomised ALERTT1 trial. The Lancet Diabetes and Endocrinology. 2023;**11**(2):96-108

[28] Sachar A, Breslin N, Ng SM. An integrated care model for mental health in diabetes: Recommendations for local implementation by the diabetes

and mental health expert working Group in England. Diabetic Medicine. 2023;**40**(4):e15029

[29] Oviedo S, Vehí J, Calm R, Armengol J. A review of personalized blood glucose prediction strategies for T1DM patients. International Journal for Numerical Methods in Biomedical Engineering. 2017;**33**(6):e2833

[30] Georga EI, Protopappas VC, Polyzos D, Fotiadis DI. Predictive modeling of glucose metabolism using free-living data of type 1 diabetic patients. Annual International Conference of the IEEE Engineering in Medicine and Biology Society. 2010;**2010**:589-592

[31] Georga EI, Protopappas VC, Polyzos D, editors. Prediction of glucose concentration in type 1 diabetic patients using support vector regression. In: Proceedings of the 10th IEEE International Conference on Information Technology and Applications in Biomedicine. Aquis Corfu Holiday Palace Hotel: IEEE; 2010. pp. 1-4

[32] Pappada SM, Cameron BD, Rosman PM, Bourey RE, Papadimos TJ, Olorunto W, et al. Neural network-based real-time prediction of glucose in patients with insulin-dependent diabetes. Diabetes Technology & Therapeutics. 2011;**13**(2):135-141

[33] Mhaskar HN, Pereverzyev SV, Walt MDvd. A deep learning approach to diabetic blood glucose prediction. Frontiers in Applied Mathematics and Statistics. 2017;**3**:14

[34] Tomczak JM. Gaussian process regression with categorical inputs for predicting the blood glucose level. In: Advances in Systems Science: Proceedings of the International Conference on Systems Science. Vol. 2017. 2016. pp. 98-108

[35] Reymann MP, Dorschky E, Eskofier BM, et. al. Blood glucose level prediction based on support vector regression using mobile platforms. In: The Conference Proceedings for the IEEE Engineering in Medicine and Biology Society. Vol. 2016. 2016. pp. 2990-2993

[36] Hidalgo JI, Colmenar JM, et al. Clarke and Parkes Error Grid Analysis of Diabetic Glucose Models Obtained with Evolutionary Computation; 2014. pp. 1305-1312

[37] Zarkogianni K, Litsa EE, Vazeou A, Nikita KS. Personalized glucose-insulin metabolism model based on self-organizing maps for patients with type 1 diabetes mellitus. In: 13th IEEE International Conference on BioInformatics and BioEngineering. 2013

[38] Woldaregay AZ, Årsand E, Walderhaug S, Albers DJ, Mamykina L, Botsis T, et al. Data-driven modeling and prediction of blood glucose dynamics: Machine learning applications in type 1 diabetes. Artificial Intelligence in Medicine. 2019;**98**:109-134

[39] Bazargani YS, Mirzaei M, Sobhi N, Abdollahi MH, Jafarizadeh A, Pedrammehr S, et al. Artificial intelligence and diabetes mellitus: An inside look through the retina. ArXiv. 2024:abs/2402.18600

[40] Vocaturo E, Zumpano E. The contribution of AI in the detection of the diabetic retinopathy. IEEE International Conference on Bioinformatics and Biomedicine (BIBM). 2020;**2020**:1516-1519

[41] Kalavar M, Al-khersan H, Sridhar J, Gorniak RJT, Lakhani P, Flanders AE, et al. Applications of artificial intelligence for the detection, management, and treatment of diabetic retinopathy. International Ophthalmology Clinics. 2020;**60**:127-145

[42] Gunasekeran DV, Ting DSW, Tan GS, Wong TY. Artificial intelligence for diabetic retinopathy screening, prediction and management. Current Opinion in Ophthalmology. 2020;**31**(5):357-365

[43] Makino M, Yoshimoto R, Ono M, Itoko T, Katsuki T, Koseki A, et al. Artificial intelligence predicts the progression of diabetic kidney disease using big data machine learning. Scientific Reports. 2019;**9**(1):11862

[44] Makino M, Ono M, Itoko T, Katsuki T, Koseki A, Kudo M, et al. Artificial intelligence predicts Progress of diabetic kidney disease-novel prediction model construction with big data machine learning. Diabetes. 2018:539

[45] Xu Q, Wang L, Sansgiry SS. A systematic literature review of predicting diabetic retinopathy, nephropathy and neuropathy in patients with type 1 diabetes using machine learning. Journal of Medical Artificial Intelligence. 2020;**3**:6

[46] Abrar SM. Artificial Intelligence for the Diagnosis and Treatment of Diabetes Kidney Disease: A Systematic Review. medRxiv. New York, USA: Cold Spring Harbor Laboratory; 2021

[47] Nallicheri A, Mahoney KM, Gutow HA, Bellini NJ, Isaacs D. Review of automated insulin delivery systems for Type 1 diabetes and associated time in range outcomes. touchREVIEWS. Endocrinology. 2022;**18**:27-34

[48] Castle JR, DeVries JH, Kovatchev BP. Future of automated insulin delivery systems. Diabetes Technology & Therapeutics. 2017;**19**(S3):S67-S72

[49] Forlenza GP, Lal RA. Current status and emerging options for automated insulin delivery systems. Diabetes Technology & Therapeutics. 2022;**24**(5):362-371

[50] Yoo JH, Kim JH. Advances in continuous glucose monitoring and integrated devices for management of diabetes with insulin-based therapy: Improvement in glycemic control. Diabetes & Metabolism Journal. 2023;**47**:27-41

[51] Klonoff DC. The artificial pancreas: How sweet engineering will solve bitter problems. Journal of Diabetes Science and Technology. 2007;**1**:72-81

[52] Thabit H, Hovorka R. Coming of age: The artificial pancreas for type 1 diabetes. Diabetologia. 2016;**59**:1795-1805

[53] Boughton CK, Hovorka R. Is an artificial pancreas (closed-loop system) for type 1 diabetes effective? Diabetic Medicine. 2018;**36**:279-286

[54] Trevitt S, Simpson S, Wood A. Artificial pancreas device systems for the closed-loop control of type 1 diabetes. Journal of Diabetes Science and Technology. 2015;**10**:714-723

[55] Nimri R, Phillip M, Clements MA, Kovatchev B. Closed-loop and artificial intelligence-based decision support systems. Diabetes Technology & Therapeutics. 2023;**25**(S1):S-89

[56] Martins IJ. Anti-aging genes improve appetite regulation and reverse cell senescence and apoptosis in global populations. Advances in Aging Research. 2016;**05**:9-26

[57] Martins IJ. Insulin therapy inactivation is connected to NAFLD and diabetes severity index. Journal of Diabetes and Clinical Studies. 2017

[58] Martins IJ. Sirtuin 1, a diagnostic protein marker and its relevance to chronic disease and therapeutic drug interventions. EC Pharmacology and Toxicology. 2018